HOW TO BE A PROFESSIONAL MAKEUP ARTIST

A Comprehensive Guide For Beginners

By: G.M. Reyna

Visit our online directory guide at www.careersinmakeup.com for links to resources mentioned in this book.

Table of Contents

Chapter 1
Makeup Artistry 101

In this Chapter you will learn:

- What is a Professional Makeup Artist?
- Exploring Makeup Styles
- The Impact of HD Technology
- Introduction to Building a Portfolio

1 What is a Professional Makeup Artist?

What is a makeup artist?

A makeup artist is someone who uses the human face and body as their canvas. They utilize makeup as a tool to diminish flaws, enhance features or totally transform an individual. You do not have to be a professional makeup artist to apply makeup. There are many who have a passion for self-expression and use makeup as a creative outlet on their leisure time. One who does for pure pleasure with no monetary compensation is often referred to as an "amateur" makeup artist.

What sets an amateur apart from a professional?

Many amateurs start applying makeup as a hobby then decide to make a career of it. However, taking it to the next level can be challenging if you're unaware of what that entails. The first step is having a clear understanding of what makes a professional a professional. So what exactly is a professional makeup artist?

It's a common belief that professional makeup artists get paid for applying makeup. And while that's true, it's important to realize that making money is only a part of it. A true professional can be defined as someone who holds high standards and strives to not only meet but exceed expectations & deliver on promises they make. Additionally, you can consider a professional as trust-worthy, consistent and a problem solver. People ultimately turn to professional makeup artists for the promise of quality, honesty and integrity.

Tips for Building a Professional Mind Set

While there is no teacher quite like experience, these helpful tips can help prepare you to think like a pro makeup artist. You'll notice most of these tips are common sense but are often overlooked by new and even experienced professionals.

Tip # 1

Practice builds confidence. Mastering the art of makeup application takes lots of practice and patience. Give yourself time to develop and fine tune your skills. Practice applying makeup on yourself and a wide variety of people (ages, complexions & ethnicities). Take your time to getting use to applying eye makeup. This area is very sensitive so extra care should be taken.

Paper makeup charts are great alternative when you do not have a real face to practice one. Not only are they inexpensive, they allow you to keep record of makeup you've done. A quick online search of "how to fill out makeup chart" will provide further instructions on how to apply and blend makeup on paper. You can find makeup charts at the following retailers:

- thefacechart.com
- amazon.com
- mudshop.com
- makeupart.net
- robertjonesbeauty.com
- paintandpowderstore.com

Another option is to use a makeup mannequin which can be reused and comes in a variety of skin tones. You can find makeup mannequins at makeupart.net.

Tip # 2

Makeup artistry is a people business. Working in makeup artistry means you're working with people. A positive attitude and a little tact can take you a long way. Strive to make a positive first impression.

Tip #3

Makeup Artistry is a visual business. In a visual business, your personal image is very important. People associate your makeup skills and professionalism with your choice of style, fashion, makeup and your overall presentation. Don't be afraid to express your individuality so long as it's done in a tasteful way.

If you're in the process of developing your personal style, you may find styling video tutorials helpful. When watching such tutorials pay attention to how stylists put together colors, prints & balance proportions. Also, take notice on how to incorporate accessories & trending items into your wardrobe (trending items are great for adding a fresh and modern element to your look). The following Youtube channels will provide you with video tutorials by professional fashion stylists:

- Chrisellelim
- Look TV
- Wendyslookbook

We also recommend the book "The Power of Style" by Bobbi Thomas, *available on bobbi.com & amazon.com.*

Tip #4

Don't skip on personal hygiene. Smelling clean is a must for any makeup artist. Nothing can make a situation more uncomfortable that bad body odor. Make sure you shower, wash your hair/body, brush your teeth, wear deodorant & so forth. Also, avoid wearing heavy perfumes that can overwhelm the person your applying makeup on. It's also important to make sure your nails are clean and kept as a reasonable length. Nails that are too long can potentially poke/scratch and cause injury.

Tip #5

Don't be shy about personal space. Many new makeup artists find it intimating to be in others' personal space or "bubble". The easiest way to overcome your fear or nerves is by practicing. Apply makeup on as many people as you can until it becomes second nature. Remember to stay calm and focus on the makeup rather than what the person is thinking.

Tip#6

Use client etiquette. A makeup session should be a relaxing experience for your customers/clients. A nice & friendly conversation helps put people at ease - avoid heated topics like politics and other sensitive subjects that can stir up strong emotions. Also, stay calm as much as you can, people sense that and will feel more comfortable themselves. It common for people to talk less when they are very relaxed, so don't feel awkward if you're not conversing 100% of the time. And last, be respectful of your client's privacy - don't post pictures of them online unless you have their permission.

Tip #7

Don't take it personal. It's impossible to please everyone. At one point in your career you will encounter a client who isn't happy with the makeup you've applied. But don't take it personal and let your feelings get hurt. Be willing to take constructive criticism with a positive attitude. See it as an opportunity to refine your skills and get better.

Tip #8

Never sacrifice your safety. Makeup artists are social creatures who are constantly meeting new people. If you ever get a creepy vibe from someone please trust your intuition and stay away from them. They may try to offer you a chance to make money but it's never worth sacrificing your safety. There will always be more opportunities!

Tip #9

Set achievable goals. Becoming a professional makeup artist doesn't happen overnight. To get where you want to go it's important to pace yourself. Take it day by day so you don't get overwhelmed. Set small goals that you reach in a realistic time frame. Check off goals as you meet them so you can track your progress.

Tip #10

Never stop learning. A career in makeup artistry is a work in progress. Even the most famous and successful makeup artists learn new techniques and ways to improve. Stay thirsty for knowledge to better yourself and expand your potential.

Publications are a great way to stay up to date and informed. Some of the most popular publications include Makeup Artist Magazine and Beauty Etc. Trade shows are another great way to learn about what's new and happening. World famous shows include IMATS, The Makeup Show & the International Beauty Show.

2 Exploring Makeup Styles

When it comes to the application of makeup, a professional makeup artist focuses on either improving or modifying the appearance of a person. Makeup used for improvement purposes is called *beauty* makeup. Makeup used for modification purposes it is referred to as *beyond beauty* makeup. In this section, you'll learn about the various styles of beauty and beyond beauty makeup.

Beauty Makeup

Beauty makeup is the most common type of makeup applied. It's used to enhance the appearance by creating symmetry and drawing attention to or away from certain features.

A professional makeup artist understands how to adapt beauty makeup to suit various skin tones, face/eye shapes and ages. To achieve this, one must have comprehensive knowledge and basic skills in the following categories:

- Color Theory
- Tools
- Skin Care
- Face
- Eyes
- Lips

Color theory involves the ability to select, combine and mix colors.

Tools include using brushes, sponges, airbrush machine, etc. for the application of face, eyes and lip makeup.

Skin care includes understanding skin types & prepping the skin for makeup with moisturizer and primer.

Face includes working with various face shapes, foundation matching & application, concealer & color correctors, setting makeup with powder, highlight & contour and applying blush & bronzer.

Eyes include working with various shapes & sizes, primer, eye shadow application, eye lining, lashes (curling, apply mascara & false lashes) and brow shaping.

Lips include shaping and color application.

Beauty Makeup Styles

There are 6 styles of beauty makeup. Within each style, makeup is applied in a way to provide a certain amount of *emphasis* or *intensity*. As you will learn in the following section, beauty styles range from soft & natural to bold & dramatic.

The 6 styles of beauty makeup include:

- Clean beauty
- Basic beauty
- Fashion
- Glamour
- Bridal/Special Occasion
- High Fashion

Clean Beauty

Also referred to as: Straight makeup and the "no makeup look"

Clean beauty refers to the way of applying makeup without the appearance of being "made up". It incorporates perfecting the skin to diminish uneven pigmentation and other flaws such as is such as blemishes, acne, scars, tattoos, birthmarks and bruises (on the face and at times the body). This also includes general grooming (shaping brushy eyebrows or unruly facial hair).

Typically, neutral colors and formulations that mimic the natural tones and texture of skin are used. This style is vitally important to compensate for the standard conditions of media productions: strong lighting, high definition cameras and in some cases distance. Overall, the main objective of clean beauty is that subjects of any race, gender or age look their very best without looking artificial. This style also serves as the basis for other beauty styles.

Basic Beauty

Also referred to as: Natural, Everyday beauty

Basic beauty begins with clean beauty but takes it a bit further by adding slightly more emphasis and definition to favorable features. Typically, soft earthy tones are used to enhance and/or add contrast in strategic places like the eyes (to make the eye color "pop"). Colors and textures also play an important role for adding a healthy glow or radiance to the skin. This style offers the wearer a polished yet fresh look that's appropriate for any occasion.

Fashion

Also referred to as: Trendy, "Latest look", is often times referred to as "glamour "makeup.

Fashion makeup begins with clean beauty then amplifies it with the use of colors, textures and shapes. Fashion makeup is inspired by pop culture (music, entertainment and fashion), women's interest magazines (fashion, celebrity gossip, beauty, etc…) as well as the runway.

Much like clothing fashion, this style recycles looks and trends from past decades - for example the "pin up look" (winged eyeliner and red lips) from the1960's or neon eye shadow from the1980's. And also like wearable fashion, what's "in" or "hot" constantly changes. Fashion looks are also influenced by cosmetic brands. Typically every season, cosmetic companies release a new ad campaign (along with a collection of makeup) - with their version of the" new must have look".

Glamour

Also referred to as: Extreme Beauty

Glamour makeup utilizes color, texture and shapes to present a subject in their most alluring and feminine way. An example of this style is seen in beauty pageant or Arabic makeup. The extreme range of Glamour can be seen in drag queen makeup - the face (and body in this case) is dramatically augmented to exude passion with a strong emphasis on sensuality.

Bridal/ Special Occasion

Also referred to as: Special event makeup, Ceremonial makeup

Bridal makeup is different for every bride. Although there are "classical looks", brides typically request a makeup look that falls within their comfort zone. It's common for someone who usually doesn't wear makeup to ask for a Basic Beauty look or "light and natural". Someone who is use to wearing makeup may want to amp it up with Glamour makeup.

In addition to a bride's personal makeup preference, the wedding theme (colors & style), cultural traditions, wedding gown and hair style are also important factors to consider. Bridal makeup can also influenced by trends found in bridal magazines & wedding planning websites as well as bridal trade shows.

Special Occasion makeup includes prom, anniversaries, graduations & other meaningful events (as well as bridal). Overall, makeup for any special occasion should begin with an understanding of how a person wants to look/feel with makeup on.

High Fashion

Also referred to as: Avant-garde, Fantasy

High Fashion makeup is considered a form of beauty makeup that's the most experimental and creative. Bold shapes, colors and textures as well as eye-catching materials like of feathers, glitter and crystals are used to create original looks. This style is commonly used in creative concept photo shoots/music videos, high fashion editorials and fashion shows. The work of Kabuki, a world renowned makeup artist, serves as a perfect example of this style.

Beyond Beauty Makeup

Beyond Beauty makeup is used to transform a performer's age, health, race, sex even species. It's used for theater, television & movie productions when an actor must look substantially different from their natural appearance to play a role.

Beyond Beauty styles include:

- Character
- Special Effects

Character Makeup

Also referred to as: Theater, Stage, Avant-garde, Fantasy

Character makeup is a technique used to enhance an actor's appearance with traditional as well as thicker cream makeup often referred to as "face and body paint" or "clown makeup". In addition to makeup, hairpieces (wigs, mustaches, beards, eyebrows) as well as molding material (wax or silicone to alter the shape of a nose for example) are used to create a character. Some performances, such the world renowned Cirque du Soleil, use character makeup in rather creative and abstract ways (referred to as "avant-garde"). Body painters are also a good example of "avant-garde" character makeup.

Other typical character makeup products include: Bald caps, body suits, dentures/teeth paint, eye contacts/drops, tears & sweat, temporary tattoos and masks.

Special Effects

Also referred to as: Special FX, Prosthetics, EMS, Gore, Trauma & 3-D makeup

Special Effects is a technique used to enhance an actor's appearance with 3-dimensional molded material or "fake skin" - also referred to as prosthetics. It can be applied to the face, head, limbs and body and is commonly used for characters that entail gory (bloody wounds, cuts, burns) or non-human attributes (monsters, creatures, aliens, etc). The process of creating prosthetics typically occurs in a makeup lab. It includes making a mold with a plaster casting (with materials such as foam, rubber, plastic, latex or gelatin). Once the mold is ready its then painted and detailed to meet the character's specifications.

There are other types of "special effects" used in productions known as Mechanical Effects and CGI (computer generated imagery). Both are considered specialized crafts and require separate training from special effects makeup.

3 The Impact of HD Technology

HD technology has significantly impacted the world of makeup artistry as well as the beauty industry. Not only has it affected the products makeup artists use, it's affected the buying choices of everyday women.

But to truly understand the impact and its affects, you must first understand what HD technology is and how it works.

In simple terms, HD technology begins with capturing a still or motion image with a HD digital camera. An HD camera is comparable to a powerful magnifying glass. In fact, it sees 6x's more clarity and detail than the human eye. Once an image is transferred to an HD screen for viewing (could be a phone screen, computer screen, TV screen or cinema screen, etc.) what your actually seeing are a multitude of tiny individual red, blue and green dots called pixels. The amount of pixels an image contains is also referred to as the 'resolution'. The higher the resolution *or higher the pixel count*, the more detailed, sharper and vibrant an image will appear.

With prior technology, known as SD Standard Definition, the resolution contained around 300,000 pixels. Images at this resolution are decent but nothing spectacular. With HD technology, the pixel count starts at around 900,000 goes as high as 3,000,000 (known as Full HD)! This significant jump in pixel count is what gives us the beautiful crystal clear images we see today.

How Have Makeup Artist Have To Adjust?

Because of the high amount of detail and clarity you get with HD, it is very unforgiving to skin imperfections as well as heavy, mismatched & unblended makeup. Makeup artists have had to adjust their skills and techniques to apply makeup that mimics the appearance of "real skin". They've come to learn a person on camera needs to look fresh and as natural as possible.

Initially, makeup that was used for HD was airbrushed on. But due to the high cost of airbrush equipment/makeup, makeup artists needed an alternative. In response to this demand, many cosmetic companies started developing makeup that provides the "airbrushed look" without the need for a machine to apply it. Although the makeup is intended for professional use, it's made available for anyone through mainstream & non-mainstream retailers. Chapter 2 - Tools of the Trade - goes into further detail about the formulation and application of HD makeup.

Thanks to social media blogs and video tutorials, information about HD makeup has spread to the masses. Everyday women are more eager to achieve the "airbrushed look" on their own. Cosmetic companies have capitalized on this by marketing HD makeup for everyday wear. The message is if it can make you look great on camera you will look even better in person.

The Future of HD Technology

Now that HD has been around for a few years technology has advanced even further. The latest cameras shoot at a resolution of 4k known as Ultra High Definition – equal to a pixel count of around 12 million! While these incredible cameras are geared towards movie and TV productions, there are 4k cameras available for consumer use. Eventually Ultra HD will become the standard just as HD has.

4 Introduction to Building a Portfolio

A portfolio is essentially a collection of images used to showcase your range of makeup skills. There are three types of portfolio formats you can choose from, they include:

- Hardcopy
- Digital
- Video

Hardcopy

This portfolio is the printed or physical version and it also referred to as your "book". Portfolios are traditionally 11x14" or 12"x15" black leather presentation binders. They are also available in a range of textures and designs. The photos that can fit in it should be at least 8.5" x 11" sized paper or bigger to really show the details of your makeup. You can even choose have it personalized with you name on the front. You can find affordable, fun & customizable portfolio binders on Zazzle.com (enter makeup artist portfolio in search bar).

Other places to buy traditional presentation binders online include: Caseenvy.com, Models-mart.com, Pinazanaro.com & Portfoliomart.com. Your local office supply store is another great place to look.

Digital

The digital version of a portfolio is seen via the internet and allows many people to view it at a low cost. You can create digital portfolio with an online website builder like moonfruit.com or wix.com. Another option is to join a social website that offers digital portfolios to their members – popular ones include modelmayhem.com, makeupart.net and bloom.com. An advantage of displaying your portfolio on a social website is having a larger audience view your portfolio. People looking for makeup services often visit social websites in search of talent.

Other popular portfolio website builders include BigBlackBag.com, Drivethrusocial.com, Foliosnap.com, Indiemade.com, Viewbook.com & Webphotomaster.com.

Video

Video is another digital version of a portfolio which can be viewed on your website or a video sharing website like Youtube.com. This option is an excellent way to get exposure to masses of people. You can easily create a video slide show of your work in minutes with online tools like animoto.com or customvideoportfolio.com.

Is building a portfolio the same for every makeup artist?

No. A makeup artist builds a portfolio to attract customers or clients within the industry/career path they work in. As you will discover later in Chapters 5-7, there are different ways to go about building a portfolio to suite the industry/career path you choose.

How much does it cost to build a portfolio?

There are two costs associated with building a portfolio. The first is the cost of the format you choose. Again, you can select from hard copy, digital and/or video. An advantage of hard copy is there is no recurring cost to display your portfolio. In other words, you only need buy a presentation binder once. However, with a hard copy portfolio there are some disadvantages. One is that you need to be physically present to show it and it can easily get lost if you're not careful. In comparison, a digital portfolio typically has recurring costs such as a monthly online subscription fee but the advantages are your portfolio can be seen on the internet 24/7 & there is no risk of it getting lost.

The other cost associated with building a portfolio is getting photos of your work. New makeup artists typically assume getting photos is an expensive task. And while it is true that hiring a photographer can be pricey, there are other ways to get images at little to no cost. Later in chapters 5-7, you'll learn more about building a portfolio in cost efficient ways to suite the industry/career path you choose.

Principals of Building a Portfolio

Whether you decide to display your portfolio in physical or digital form, there are 4 principals every makeup artist should remember:

Principal #1

Quality is more important that quantity. 5-10 amazing pictures is will represent you better as a makeup artist that 30 so-so images.

Principal # 2

A portfolio should show your range of makeup skills. A great way to do this is by applying different makeup styles on the same person. This will show your ability to enhance the same features in different ways. Also consider women of different nationalities, skin colors and face/eye shapes.

Principal #3

Keep your portfolio organized – group similar categories of makeup styles/looks together. You may consider showing all the natural looks first, then fashion looks and then perhaps glamour looks. The idea is to create a flow for the viewer.

Principal #4

A portfolio is a work in progress. As your makeup skills improve over time, your portfolio should reflect that.

Chapter 2
Tools of the Trade

In This Chapter:

- Professional vs. Budget Makeup
- Airbrush Makeup Q & A
- Understanding HD Makeup
- Building a Kit Part 1: What's in a Kit?
- Building a Kit Part 2: Other Helpful Advice

5 Professional vs. Budget Makeup

Much like a fine chef, a professional makeup artist relies on high-quality ingredients to deliver high-quality results. In makeup artistry, "high-quality" refers to makeup that is <u>strongly pigmented,</u> easy to blend and can endure many hours of wear under a variety of conditions (for example, hot studio lights or humid climates). In addition to adequate coverage and longevity, professional makeup also meets the needs of makeup artists in the areas of color selection, texture and finish.

A great benefit of professional makeup is that is it very cost effective. Although it does cost more than makeup you find at the drugstore, it last substantially longer. A little goes a long way and this saves you money over time. Another advantage is that is increases your credibility because professional makeup is associated with quality & prestige.

Professional makeup can be purchased through "mainstream" and "non-mainstream" retailers. In the next section, we'll discuss the differences as well as the advantages & disadvantages of each retail channel. And later in Chapter 2-What's In A Kit?- you'll learn how to get the best deals and how to avoid costly mis-purchases when buying makeup for your kit.

Mainstream Professional Makeup

Mainstream professional is also referred to as *prestige, luxury, premium or high-end makeup*. Mainstream makeup brands are well known to the general public. Examples of popular mainstream brands include MAC, Smashbox & Urban Decay.

You can purchase pro mainstream makeup in-store or online through major mass retailers like Sephora. You can also find it at exclusive online retailers, fine department stores, makeup brand websites & wholesale makeup outlets.

Advantages of Mainstream Makeup

- Most in store retailers have makeup artist/beauty advisors that provide assistance and can answer questions you may have.

- Testers are typically provided at in-store retailers – lets you test out makeup before you buy.

- Retailers generally have an open return policy. If you change your mind after opening and using a product, you return it for a full refund.

- Many retailers offer free samples of makeup with purchase.

- Most makeup brands and retailers offer discounts to professional makeup artists.

- Makeup is often made in travel and sample sizes- give you a chance to try at lower cost.

- Amazing deals and discounts around the holidays

Disadvantages of Mainstream Makeup

- Retail markup can be high

- Colors/products can be discontinued without notice

Non-mainstream Professional Makeup

Non-mainstream professional makeup refers to makeup brands that design their products with the makeup artist in mind. They cater to the needs of professional makeup artists with an extensive variety of palettes and other products that are packaged for easy portability. Because non-mainstream brands do not advertise to the masses, they aren't very popular or well known among the general public. Some non-mainstream professional brands include Ben Nye, Mehron & Graftobian.

Non-mainstream professional makeup is sold through authorized dealers. Authorized dealers can be found online or locally. Popular online dealers include Cinemasecrets.com, Naimes.com and Camerareadycosmetics.com. Local dealers include beauty supply stores, beauty salons and some seasonal costume shops. Makeup shows such as IMATS & IBS are another popular outlet to purchase non-mainstream makeup.

In addition to offering traditional beauty makeup aka *straight makeup*, many non-mainstream dealers also supply theatrical and special-fx makeup.

Advantages of Non-mainstream Makeup

- Retail mark up is often lower than mainstream makeup
- Geared towards all types of professional makeup artists
- Most brands offer professional makeup artist discounts
- Products are generally not discontinued without notice as much as mainstream makeup.

Disadvantage of Non-mainstream Makeup

- Not as widely or locally available as mainstream makeup
- Some local dealers may require you to have a cosmetology/esthetics license to purchase.

What's the difference between professional makeup & "budget" makeup?

Budget makeup is also called *drugstore, thrift or mass production* makeup. It costs substantially less that professional makeup because it's made with lower quality ingredients & is less pigmented. Some popular budget brands include Avon, Eyes Lips Face (ELF) & Wet n' Wild.

Budget makeup can be purchased through discount retail stores such as Wal-Mart, Target and dollar stores. It's also available through local drugstores, grocery stores and other retailers that sell beauty and health related products. In addition, you can buy budget makeup through direct sales channels like Avon and Mary Kay as well as on websites that cater to makeup enthusiasts like coastalscents.com, bhcosmetics.com, eyeslipsface.com and cherryculture.com.

Advantages of budget makeup

- Affordable & widely available
- Find deals as low as $.99
- Large selection of colors & palettes
- Good to practice without breaking the bank

Disadvantages of budget makeup

- Budget brands do not offer Professional Artist Discounts
- Most stores have strict refund polices and will not let you return the makeup if you've used it and changed your mind.
- Has a reputation of being "cheap" & "ineffective".
- Some eye shadows can be extremely powdery & won't show up without a good base or primer.

Although the disadvantages seem to outweigh the advantages of budget makeup, many cosmetic companies are working on changing that. You see, in the last several years a new trend has emerged in the budget makeup market. More and more budget brands are focused on adding more value by reformulating their products with newer and better ingredients. More attention has also gone into color selection and the packaging to deliver a "high-end" look that resembles expensive professional brands. The "high-end" look at "low-end" prices has developed into a trend referred to as "masstige" (which is basically the combination of "mass production" and "prestige"). Popular brands that have jumped on the "masstige" trend include Wet n'Wild, NYX Cosmetics and Eyes Lips Face's Studio Line.

6   Airbrush Makeup Q & A

New makeup artists often find airbrushing to be complicated subject but it doesn't have to be. To assist you in making informed decisions about this medium, we've answered some of the most frequently asked questions.

Q) What is airbrush makeup?

A) Airbrush makeup is thin highly pigmented liquid that can be used on the face and body. It's applied with an air-operated device called an airbrush machine. The airbrush machine system consists of air source/compressor, an air hose that connects the compressor and an airbrush gun.
The airbrush gun allows makeup artists to disperse a fine mist of microscopic dots evenly & lightly on the skin.

Q) When did makeup artists start using airbrush makeup?

A) Records show airbrush makeup was used on a movie set back in1925.

Q) What are some of the advantages of using airbrush makeup?

A) Because of its thin but opaque formula, airbrush makeup can be applied lightly yet still offer full coverage. It provides the look of naturally "flawless" skin that's never heavy or cakey. It also last long on the skin and is durable in a variety of climates. Some formulas are also sweat and waterproof.

Airbrush makeup is suitable and compatible with HD technology.

Many makeup artists prefer to use airbrush makeup because it is sanitary. With airbrush you do not have to touch the skin so helps prevent spreading bacteria.

Q) What are some of the disadvantages of using airbrush makeup?

A) Touch ups can be difficult if you cannot carry the machine with you. Most makeup artists have to use traditional makeup and tools (brushes and sponges) for touch ups.

Airbrush makeup and equipment is considered a special product and can be costly.

Q) Where can I get the best deals on airbrush makeup?

A) When shopping for airbrush makeup, look for professional kits and value packs to save money. Some kits contain a range of makeup shades as well as the airbrush machine. Some sell the airbrush machine separately. Another great way to save money is by buying sample or "mini" sizes rather than full size bottles of makeup. Great places to find airbrush kits/value packs, equipment and accessories include:

- Amazon.com
- Camerareadycosmetics.com
- Dinair.com
- Graftobian.com
- Kettcosmetics.com
- Love-makeup.co.uk
- Luminessair.com
- Makeupdesignory.com
- Naimies.com
- Occmakeup.com
- Paintandpowderstore.com

- Temptupro.com

Many of these online stores offer up to 30% off their products to professional makeup artists as well as students. It might be worth waiting to qualify for a discount before you invest in airbrush makeup. For specific details visit each store and look for "Pro Artist Discount" or "Pro".

Q) How can I learn to apply airbrush makeup?

A) There are many resources available that will teach you how to properly apply airbrush makeup. You may consider attending a course at a makeup school. You can find how-to videos and information about workshops at:

- Dinair.com
- Kettcosmetics.com
- Luminessair.com
- OCCmakeup.com
- Temptupro.com

We also recommend:

- Temptu Airbrush Makeup 101 DVD

Q) What else should I know about airbrushing?

A) Airbrush equipment and the airbrush gun must be cleaned so it can evenly disperse the makeup. You'll need to make sure you have an airbrush cleaning kit made especially for your airbrush system.

Airbrush systems must be plugged into an electric outlet. Make sure the machine's plug will fit into your country's standard outlet.

ADDITIONAL RESOURCES

Suzanne Patterson is an Emmy award winning makeup artist who specializes in airbrushing. She's had decades of experience in movies &television working with some of the biggest stars in the Hollywood like Arnold Schwarzenegger, Queen Latifah, Jennifer Love Hewitt & many other celebrities. Suzanne shares her expertise and offers free valuable advice on her blog creativeartistryfx.com/blog. For information about airbrush classes and workshops by Suzanne visit creativeartistryfx.com.

7 Understanding HD Makeup

HD makeup is lightweight and highly pigmented. When properly applied in thin layers, it's unnoticeable or "invisible" on the skin. But although the application is very light, the concentration of pigment provides medium to full coverage. The end result is even and flawless skin that looks incredibly "real".

In addition to being lightweight and highly pigmented, HD makeup contains fine light reflecting particles that give the skin a delicate luminous sheen. The particles also work to blur the appearance fine lines, pores, blemishes and other imperfections. The effect is commonly referred to as "soft focus" or "photo ready".

What does HD compatible mean?

HD compatible refers to makeup that delivers the same results as HD makeup. Airbrush makeup is considered HD compatible.

Who makes HD makeup?

Many mainstream & non-mainstream professional brands produce HD makeup. Popular brands include:

Mainstream

- Makeup Forever
- NARS
- Smashbox

Non-mainstream

- Ben Nye
- Eve Pearl
- Graftobian

- Kryolan
- Mehron

As consumer awareness & demand for HD makeup increases, budget brands are responding by bringing affordable HD products to the market. Although there is only a handful of HD budget makeup right now, there's no doubt we'll see more in the near future. Popular brands include:

- E.L.F.
- NYX
- LA Girl

The Future of HD Makeup

As HD technology continues to advance, so will the makeup. Popular brands like Urban Decay are already creating weightless "ultra definition" makeup to meet the high standards of "razor sharp" Ultra HD technology.

Additional Resources

To learn more about HD makeup application we recommend the following DVD:

HD Makeup 101 - Achieving Perfection with Simplicity by Graftobian

8 Building a Kit Part 1: What's In a Kit?

A professional makeup kit is composed of three categories: makeup, tools and equipment. Within each category, there are sub-categories as follows:

Makeup:

- makeup
- storage

Tools:

- brushes
- brush storage
- makeup hygiene
- accessories
- disposables
- preparation

Equipment

- light
- mirror
- chair

MAKEUP

There are 3 types of makeup:

- Beauty
- Character
- Special FX

Beauty *also known straight makeup* is the most common makeup used across all fields of makeup artistry. It includes makeup for the eyes, lips and face. Common items include:

- *Eyes:* Moisturizer, primer, eye shadow, liner, mascara, lash curler, false lashes & eyebrow pencils/powders

- *Lips:* Moisturizer, primer, lipstick, gloss & stains

- *Face:* Moisturizer, primer, concealer/corrector, foundation, setting powder, cheek color, highlighter & bronzer

Character makeup is used for theater, TV and movie productions and includes such items as cream makeup, face and body paint, molding material, stage blood, dentures/teeth paint, eye contacts/drops, tears & sweat, adhesive and adhesive removers, beards, moustaches, wigs, bald caps, temporary tattoos and tattoo cover up.

Special FX makeup is also used for theater, TV and movie productions and includes liquid latex, cream makeup to simulate bruises and other trauma, fake blood, scars, sweat & tears.

Building Your Makeup Collection

The quickest & most cost efficient way to build a makeup collection is by purchasing palettes travel/sample sizes & value-kits/sets. When shopping for a value set/kit, be sure to do a price comparison between the cost of a set/kit and the cost of buying products individually. Sometimes, it can be less expensive to purchase makeup separately rather than buying a pre-customized set.

Also, when building your collection, don't be afraid to mix and match makeup brands. Rarely will you ever see a professional makeup kit with only one brand.

How to get the best deals on makeup

Makeup outlets offer up to 75% discount on budget and professional makeup that is considered overstock, discontinued or factory blemished. Visit these makeup outlets for great deals at rock bottom prices:

- Allcosmeticswholesale.com
- Dextermakeup.com
- BeautyCrunch.com
- CherryCulture.com
- Suite7beauty.com

Popular in-store makeup outlets include Nordstrom Rack, Marshall's, TJ Maxx, Estee Lauder CCO & Ross.

Take advantage of pro discounts (up to 40%) offered by professional makeup brands and retailers. In "Building a Kit Part 2" you can learn more about pro artist discounts programs.

Shop the sales and clearance section online or in-stores. Stay informed about what's on sale or clearance by signing up for a store's mailer/advertisement. Also, look for retailers that offer reward points for shopping with them. Reward points can be typically redeemed for free makeup products or discounts on future purchases.

Don't be shy to ask for free samples when shopping in-store. Sales reps at department stores and retailers like Sephora are happy to give samples to bring customers back.

Shop during the holidays. Almost all retailers offer amazing bargains on value sets meant to be offered as gifts.

When shopping online look for coupon codes & free shipping deals. You can find discounts codes for most online retailers at retailmenot.com.

Attend trade shows like IMATS or IBS to buy professional makeup at discounted promotional prices.

Where to Shop for Makeup

Below you'll find a list of retailers where you can shop for mainstream and non-mainstream professional makeup as well as budget makeup. To link to these retailers, visit our online directory guide at careersinmakeup.com & click on Shop Makeup, Tools & Equipment.

Where to buy Mainstream Professional Makeup

Bobbibrowncosmetics.com, Benefitcosmetics.com, Esteelauder.com, Lauramercier.com, Loraccosmetics.com, MACcosmetics.com, MakeupForever.com, Narscosmetics.com, Smashbox.com, Toofaced.com, Tartecosmetics.com, Thebalm.com, Stilacosmetics.com, Urbandecay.com

You can also shop for an assortment of mainstream brands at these retailers:

- Amazon.com
- Beautyhabit.com
- Beso.com
- Bloom.com
- Gurumakeupemporium.com
- HSN.com
- Marketamerica.com
- QVC.com
- Sephora.com
- Ulta.com
- Zappos.com

Where to buy Non-Mainstream Professional Makeup

Bennye.com, Camerareadycosmetics.com, Cinemasecrets.com, CoverFX.com, Evepearl.com, Faceatelier.com, Graftobian.com,

Inglotcosmetics.com, Kryolan.com, LaFemmecosmetics.com, Mehron.com, MUDshop.com, RCMAmakeup.net, Viseart.com, Yabycosmetics.com, Threecustom.com

You can also shop for an assortment of non-mainstream brands at these authorized dealers:

- Alconeco.com
- Amazon.com
- Ballbeauty.com
- Beautydive.com
- Cosplaysupplies.com
- Frendsbeautysupplyonline.com
- Lecosmetique.com
- Makeupart.net
- Mallatts.com
- Megamakeupstore.com
- Naimies.com
- Preciousaboutmakeup.com
- Rickysnyc.com
- Sigmabeauty.com
- Starsmakeuphaven.com

Where to buy Budget makeup

If you're on a budget and need more affordable makeup options, check out these discount retailers:

- Allcosmeticswholesale.com
- Avon.com
- Beautydive.com
- BHCosmetics.com
- Coastalscents.com
- Cherryculture.com
- Eyeslipsface.com
- Forever21.com

- Jordanacosmetics.com
- Lightinthebox.com
- Milanicosmetics.com
- Makeupgeek.com
- Meetmark.com
- NYXcosmetics.com
- Rubykissescosmetics.com
- Sallybeauty.com
- Shanycosmetics.com
- Sleekmakeup.com
- Target.com
- Tmart.com
- Victoriassecret.com
- Walgreens.com
- Walmart.com

Makeup Storage

When it comes to makeup storage, you can choose from:

- Soft bags
- Hard cases w/out lights
- Hard cases w/lights
- Soft cases
- With or w/out wheels

Before you start shopping for makeup storage, consider these important factors:

Dimension
How much total space does it take up? If you need to fly with it will it fit in the overhead compartment of the plane or will it need to be flown separately risking it being damaged or lost? How much makeup do you have and how big does the storage bag/case need to be to fit it all?

Accessibility

If for some reason a workspace surface is not available would you be able to work out of the storage bag/case? Can you find what you need easily?

Compartments

How many compartments does it have? Will it suit the way you would like to organize your makeup?

Portability

Is it easy to take with you? If it has wheels, do they turn smoothly?

Weight

How much does the storage bag/case weigh before adding the weight of the makeup? If you need to travel, will the total weight make it strenuous on you?

Lighting

Do you need a consistent light source? Will you be traveling and need to have control of the lighting conditions?

Where to shop for makeup cases and storage

Below is a list of resources where you can find a variety of makeup storage options to suit your needs & budget. To link to these retailers, visit careersinmakeup.com & click on Shop Makeup, Tools & Equipment.

- Alconeco.com
- Caboodle.com
- EvePearl.com
- FaceStockholm.com
- Frendsbeautysupplyonline.com
- Glamcor.com
- GuruMakeupEmporium.com
- HarmonDiscount.com

- Japonesque.com
- KettCosmetics.com
- Lecosmetique.com
- Makeupart.net
- Naimies.com
- NYXcosmetics.com
- PaintandPowderstore.com
- PowderGroup.com
- Preciousaboutmakeup.com
- Sephora.com
- Shanycosmetics.com
- SoniaKashuk.com
- Target.com
- Thekimgreeneline.com
- Thepromakeupshop.com
- Walmart.com
- Yazmo.com
- Zuca.com

KIT TOOLS

Brushes

Much like makeup, brushes are also recognized as professional or budget grade. When choosing brushes, it's preferable that you go with professional grade for several reasons. First of all, professional brushes are made with higher quality materials as well as construction. Although professional brushes will you cost you more than budget/ drugstore brushes, they are far more durable & resistant to water damage. Generally you can expect to get 2-10 years of use (that includes daily use and frequent cleanings).

Budget or *drugstore* brushes cost a fraction of the price of professional brushes. In fact, you can find brushes as low as $1.00 (visit eyeslipsface.com) Its important to remember, that while you may be getting a great bargain with budget brushes, you cannot to expect them to endure the same wear and tear that professional brushes can. It doesn't take a lot for a budget brush to come apart, so you have to be extra careful when using, storing and cleaning them.

Building Your Brush Collection

The quickest way to build your brush collection is to purchase value sets. It's important however, to do a price comparison between the cost of a set vs. buying individual brushes. Sometimes, it can be less expensive to purchase brushes separately for eyes, lips and face rather than buying a pre-customized set.

If your purchasing brushes individually, it's definitely ok to mix and match brands. It's very common for a professional makeup artist to have a brush collection that includes various brands at various price points.

General rules of thumb when it comes to brushes:

- Look for brushes with <u>soft</u> bristles to avoid scratching and irritating the skin. Remember, the finer the bristles/hair the smoother the application will be.

- Dense or *tightly-packed* bristles deposit a strong amount of color.

- Fluffy & *less-compacted* bristles deposit color lightly for more of a hazy or diffused effect.

- Synthetic bristles are non-absorbent. They work well with liquid, cream and powder makeup.

- Natural animal hair bristles are absorbent and tend to work best dryer makeup like creams and powders.

How to care for your brushes

You can extend the life of your brushes by following these easy storage and cleaning tips:

- Store your brushes properly so the bristles stay in shape. The most popular storage options include roll-up pouch, brush belt or brush holder/cup.

- Keep brushes clean and free of contamination by using brush sanitizer after each use. You'll also want to give your brushes regular deep cleanings to remove traces of any makeup build-up. To deep clean your brushes you can use either a brush shampoo or mild soap like baby shampoo. Be sure to condition afterwards with a mild hair conditioner to keep the bristles soft and healthy.

- Never stand a wet brush upright! Water or cleanser can seep into the ferrule and break up the glue that holds the bristles. Always lay the brush flat to dry on a clean surface.

- When you first purchase brushes, you may notice the bristles "shedding" a little. Washing your brushes before using them for the first time can help reduce shedding

- When you wash your brushes for the first time, you may notice a black or inky color which is simply dye from the bristles. After a few washes, you should see less dye.

Where to shop for makeup brushes

Almost every professional mainstream, non-mainstream and budget makeup brand/retailer sells brushes. There are literally thousands of places you can shop, so to help you we've gathered a list of popular and trusted online retailers. To link to these retailers, visit careersinmakeup.com & click on Shop Makeup, Tools & Equipment.

Choose from a wide selection of professional grade brushes at these online retailers.

- Allcosmeticswholesale.com
- Ballbeauty.com
- Bdellium.com
- Crownbrush.com
- Makeupart.net
- Maccosmetics.com
- Naimies.com
- Rickysnyc.com
- Royalbrush.com
- Smashbox.com
- Sephora.com
- Sigma.com
- Ulta.com

If you're looking for more affordable options, check out these budget retailers:

- BHcosmetics.com
- Coastalscents.com
- Eyeslipsface.com
- Meetmark.com
- Shanycosmetics.com
- Soniakashuk.com

In addition to these retailers, art supply stores are also a great place to look for brushes. While they are necessarily sold as "makeup brushes" they are generally constructed the same way and are safe to use.

Brush Storage

Storing your brushes properly will help maintain the original shape of the bristles thus extending their overall lifetime usage. It also assists you in staying organized so you can be more effective and productive. The storage unit you decide on will directly reflect the method that you like to work. You can choose from:

- Brush roll/wrap
- Brush belt/apron
- Brush holder/cup

A **brush rolls/wraps** works best if you like having the brushes laid out in front of you so you can see them all at a glance.

A **brush belt/apron** may suit you if you like having the brushes close to you so you don't have to reach out for them.

A **brush holder/cup** works well if you prefer for your brushes standing upright so you can easily reach for them.

Below you'll find list of online retailers where you can find these brush storage options. To link to these retailers visit careersinmakeup.com & click on Shop Makeup, Tools & Equipment.

- BeautyDive.com
- CameraReadyCosmetics.com
- EvePearl.com
- Eyeslipsface.com
- Frendsbeautysupplyonline.com
- GuruMakeupEmporium.com
- Inglotcosmetics.com
- MakeupMag.com
- Nyxcosmetics.com
- RoyalBrushStore.com
- Shanycosmetics.com
- Sigmabeauty.com
- Yazmo.com

Kits Tools: Makeup Hygiene

One of the most important aspects of being a professional makeup artist is being considerate of your customers/clients' health and well being. The following products will help ensure you are reducing the risk of spreading harmful bacteria, infection and disease. Makeup hygiene & sanitation products include:

- Hand Sanitizer
- Brush Cleaner
- Makeup Antibacterial Spray
- Disinfection Products *

*Disinfection products should be used to disinfect makeup packaging as well as brush handles and equipment. You can choose to use either disposable wipes or a reusable UV light like the Zadro Nano UV Disinfection Light.

Please Note: They majority of hygiene & sanitation products contain alcohol which can cause a burning or irritating sensation. Be sure to wait until these products have dried completely before you make contact with your guest - especially around the eye area!

You can find makeup hygiene, sanitation products and more information at the following online retailers. To link to these retailers, visit careersinmakeup.com & click on Shop Makeup, Tools & Equipment.

- Beautysoclean.com
- Thepromakeupshop.com
- Safebeautyassociation.com
- Alconeco.com

Accessories

Accessories include miscellaneous items that a makeup artist often reaches for:

- **Color wheel** for selecting and combining colors.
- **Face charts** to record makeup looks or for practice.
- **Rubbing Alcohol** to fix broken powder makeup.
- **Empty palettes** for mixing or transferring/organizing individual products (lipstick, eye shadows, blushes, etc…)

Disposables

In addition to hygiene & sanitation products, disposables are essential to help eliminate the spread of bacteria. Disposable products include:

- Mascara wands
- Lip color wands
- Q-tips
- Cotton Balls
- Sponges
- Makeup wipes
- Spatulas*
- Palette*

*Spatulas are used to remove products from its container in a hygienic way. Makeup is then transferred to a palette for mixing & application. Most pro makeup artists choose to use reusable stainless steel spatula/ palette. If you decide to use a metal spatula/palette make sure to disinfect it after each use.

You can find disposable products at your local drugstore or beauty supply store. If you wish to shop online, here is a list of retailers that carry disposable products. To link to these retailers, visit careersinmakeup.com & click on Shop Makeup, Tools & Equipment.

- Naimies.com
- Makeupart.net

- Thepromakeupshop.com
- Alconeco.com
- Auralinebeauty.com
- Ebay.com

Preparation

Before you begin a makeup application it's important to protect your guest clothes from makeup stains and other potential disasters. Preparation also includes getting hair out the way so you work comfortably.

Preparation tools include:

- Cape
- Hair clips

It's important to keep your preparation tools clean. Make sure you wash your cape often and you wash hairclips with hot water and soap. If you don't want to spend time constantly washing hair clips, you may consider using elastic bands and bobby pins which are cheap and disposable.

KIT EQUIPMENT

Kit Equipment: Light

The best (and free) light source you can find is daylight. Natural sunlight is actually white and lets you see the true colors of skin and makeup. Whenever possible try doing makeup by a window where light is being filtered through a sheer white curtain. If daylight is not available be aware that common household and commercial light bulbs produce a variety of hues that affect the way you see the true skin tones and the color of the makeup being applied. Below are some examples of common light bulbs and the color hue they produce:

- **Fluorescent** light produces a Greenish-Blue hue

- **Halogen** light produces a Slightly Warm Yellow-Red hue

- **Warm White** light produces a Warm Yellow-Red hue

- **Incandescent** light produces a very Warm Yellow-Red

Whenever you need to use an artificial light source, make sure the bulbs are blue (otherwise known as full spectrum light bulbs). Blue light bulbs mimic sunlight/natural light because the color they cast is white.

If you have the advantage of working at a makeup station with a mirror and vanity lights, be sure that the light bulbs installed are again *full spectrum light bulbs*. If you are interested in a stationary makeup vanity/station that comes ready with full spectrum lights check out:

- VanityGirlHollywood.com
- Glamcor.com

If you find that you need a light source that you can travel with, a great option would be to purchase either a portable makeup station (which comes with a built in mirror and vanity lights) or a standalone lighting system. You can find makeup cases/stations with lights at the following online retailers. To link to these retailers, visit careersinmakeup.com & click on Shop Makeup, Tools & Equipment.

- Amazon.com
- Frendsbeautysupplyonline.com
- Glamcor.com
- Lecosmetique.com
- Makeupart.net
- NYXCosmetics.com
- PaintandPowderstore.com

- Preciousaboutmakeup.com
- Shanycosmetics.com

You can find stand alone lighting systems at these retailers:

- Glamcor.com
- PaintandPowderstore.com
- Preciousaboutmakeup.com

Please note: Sometimes light bulbs for any of these light sources are sold separately. Be sure to double check the product description for more details.

Kit Equipment: Mirror

The type of mirror you need depends on where you plan to apply makeup. A traveling makeup artist may find it easy to carry a hand held mirror or have a makeup case that comes with one. A stationary makeup artist may consider mounting a mirror on the wall or look for a vanity with a built in mirror.

Kit Equipment: Chair

Nothing can be more exhausting and back straining than consistently being hunched over to apply makeup on someone. When it comes to chairs, find one that so when your guest sits down they are at eye level with you. The chair should also have a back rest and be comfortable.

Director's chairs are often used as makeup chairs. You can also find chairs specifically geared towards makeup artists. These chairs are popular mainly because they are padded for extra comfort & many of them have a side table for extra workspace and/or side pockets for extra storage space. These types of chairs are also great if you travel as they are lightweight and portable.

If you're interested in a makeup chair, you can find one at the following online suppliers. To link to these retailers, visit careersinmakeup.com & click on Shop Makeup, Tools & Equipment.

- EvePearl.com
- Frendsbeautysupplyonline.com
- PaintandPowderStore.com
- MakeupArt.net
- Preciousaboutmakeup.com
- Naimies.com
- Shanycosmetics.com

9 Building a Kit Part 2: Helpful Advice & Tips

Save up to 40% off on makeup, tools and equipment

Many professional mainstream & non-mainstream brands/retailers offer discount programs to professional makeup artists. Whenever possible, take advantage of these discounts which can save you up to 40% off on makeup, tools and equipment for your kit.

Popular brands that offer such discounts include MAC Cosmetics, Smashbox & Makeup Forever. You can find out about their discount programs by visiting their website and clicking on or searching for "Pro Membership". Typically, companies will ask for credentials that prove you're a professional makeup artist such as your website, business card or more. If you plan to attend a makeup or beauty school, you may qualify for a "student discount".

You can find the links to the above mentioned makeup brands and others that offer discount programs at careersinmakeup.com.

Find out what others are saying

A little online research can help you make informed decisions about products you may want to purchase. You can find reviews by conducting an online search (name of product here) + reviews. You can also check out the following makeup community websites for consumer reviews:

- Makeupalley.com
- Inmykit.com
- Temptalia.com
- Makeupgeek.com
- Youtube.com *

If you cannot find the reviews you are looking for, consider joining a forum or a board (most of these sites have forums/boards). There you can ask others if they have any experience with particular products. You'd be surprised to find how tight-knit the makeup community is. They are very willing to help and even make recommendations..

*There has been talk within the YouTube makeup community of un-honest "paid" reviews. To protect yourself don't rely on one review alone. Look for more videos and/or use the other review websites to get a few opinions.

Keep Your Kit Tidy

A clean & well organized kit lets you client know you value their health & well being. A dirty kit can speak volumes and may send the wrong message about you.

Protect Your Kit

After investing so much money on your kit, wouldn't it be a shame if it was damaged, lost or stolen? Kit insurance can offer you piece of mind in case of an unfortunate event. Learn more at imakeupmatters.com.

Chapter 3
Education & Training

In This Chapter:

- Makeup Artist Licensing
- Beauty School vs. Makeup School
- How to Choose a Makeup School
- Alternative Learning Tools & Training Resources
- The Little Black Book of Celebrity Makeup Artists

10   Makeup Artist Licensing

In every US state, there is a Board of Cosmetology that regulates laws and regulations concerning public health/safety in connection with beauty practices. These laws are essentially created to control and prevent the spread of infection/disease. Beauty professionals (hairdressers, nail techs, and estheticians, etc.) working with chemicals are required to abide by these laws in all 50 US states.

In certain states, cosmetology boards have included makeup artists to their list of beauty professionals. While they understand a makeup artist doesn't work with chemicals, they feel they are just as liable to spread infection/disease with contaminated brushes & makeup.

To ensure a person is capable of working safely with the public, they are required to pass an exam issued by the state's cosmetology board. If they pass, they are issued a Cosmetology License. If they do not pass, they will not be issued a license and can be penalized if they are found working without one.

In order to take the cosmetology exam you must first complete a cosmetology program at a beauty school. A cosmetology program covers hair, skin and nails and provides training in proper sanitation, disinfection and hygiene procedures (commonly referred to as "safe beauty" or "beauty hygiene" procedures). It also teaches how recognize the signs of disease to avoid putting your own health at risk. Once you've completed the program, you can then take the cosmetology exam.

Once you obtain a license you can begin working. To keep your license current and in good standing, you'll have to pay a renewal fee which is typically due every year.

The Pros and Cons of Cosmetology Programs

Cosmetology programs do have their advantages as well disadvantages. On one hand, with a cosmetology license you can style hair and do nails along with applying makeup. But, on the other hand, cosmetology programs can last a year or longer and can cost several thousand dollars. They also tend to put a bigger emphasis on hair & nails than skin (which covers makeup application.) A 1 year program may only cover makeup for about 3 weeks!

If a cosmetology program is required but doesn't sound right for you, generally a safe alternative for a makeup artist is an esthetics program (also offered at beauty schools). In an esthetics program, you would learn a lot more about makeup since the entire curriculum is based on the science of skin. And since it takes a lot less time to complete, it saves you both time and money. After finishing the program, you'll be required to pass the Cosmetology Board's exam to get an Esthetics License.

Will You Need a License?

To determine if you will need a license, start by contacting your state's Cosmetology Board or local beauty school. The question you'll need them to answer is "do I need to pass a cosmetology (or esthetics) exam to do makeup"? They may ask you what career path you're interested in as this can affect the answer.

Word of caution: Beauty schools may say licensing is required just to get you to enroll. It's recommend that you call several schools to see if you get the same response. If you get mixed answers, contact your state's Cosmetology Board to be 100% sure.

The Next Step

If a license IS required...

If your Cosmetology Board says a license is required, start researching beauty schools in your area that fit within your budget and lifestyle. Many schools offer full or part time classes, even night classes as well as financial aid if you qualify. See Resources below to find schools in your area.

If a license is NOT required...

If a license is not required, you'll still need to educate yourself in disease control and prevention or "safe beauty". You have several options to do this. You may consider taking a cosmetology/esthetics program or attend a makeup school that focuses on makeup hygiene. You can also find many articles as well as video tutorials online. There are also books that provide full cosmetology/esthetics training or just general makeup hygiene (see Resources below for more info).

Please Note: Finishing a book on cosmetology doesn't mean you could take a Cosmetology exam for a license. In order to take the exam, you are required to complete an accredited cosmetology program.

Please Take this Information Seriously!!

It's important to understand that whether it's enforced by the law or not, a professional makeup artist is responsible for the health & safety of others. Learning to following safe beauty procedures is a fundamental part of your training. While you may be eager to start doing makeup, do not overlook this matter. Unwanted legal complications like lawsuits or disciplinary action by the State Board of Cosmetology can result from ignoring this!

ADDITIONAL RESOURCES

Safe Beauty Association

The Safe Beauty Association is dedicated to educating, informing and bring awareness about makeup hygiene. Their website safebeautyassociation.com provides a wealth of information.

Beauty So Clean

Visit Youtube channel beautysoclean for video tutorials on sanitizing makeup and brushes. Their website beautysoclean.com is also filled with valuable information.

Books on cosmetology, aesthetics & makeup hygiene:

- Milady Standard Cosmetology 2012 by Milady
- Milady Standard Esthetics: Fundamentals by Milady
- The Professional Makeup Artist by Vincent Blasco and Vincent J-R Kehoe
- Make-Up Designory's Beauty Make-Up by Yvonne Hawker

Find a cosmetology/aesthetics program in your area visit:

- BeautySchoolsDirectory.com
- MySocialBeauty.com
- Beautyandcosmetologyschools.com

11 Beauty School vs. Makeup School

What is difference between beauty school & makeup school?

Beauty schools offer cosmetology, esthetics and nail programs. These programs specifically train you in disease control and prevention procedures. In a cosmetology program you learn about working with hair, skin and nails. An esthetics programs just teaches about skin. When you complete either program & pass an exam issued by the State Board you receive either a cosmetology or aesthetics license.

While beauty school is a step in the right direction, it may not provide you with all the training you need to begin a career path in makeup artistry. We strongly encourage you to consider makeup school or alternative learning tools/training to expand your knowledge & skills.

Makeup schools provide specialized courses that focus on particular styles of makeup application (for example – beauty, bridal, special effects, film, etc.) After completing a course, you receive either a certificate or diploma. Either document serves as proof that you completed the course. The value of a cert. or diploma is determined by the credibility of the school and your instructors.

What Is The Difference Between A License And A Diploma/Certificate?

Certificates & diplomas are NOT the same as licenses. Diplomas and certificates tell more about your makeup skills, a license is about proving professional credibility. Licenses are issued by the State Board of Cosmetology after passing a cosmetology exam. It is actually a legal document.

12   How to Choose a Makeup School

Makeup schools and academies offer a variety of specialized courses. Some courses are designed help you build skills specific to your career path in addition to teaching makeup application techniques. Others focus only on makeup application techniques.

One of the greatest benefits of a makeup school is that you have an instructor to guide you and answer questions you may have. It also consists of a structured learning plan that specifies what topics must be understood.

A disadvantage of a makeup school can be the price. Courses can run between hundred to several thousand dollars. Because it is such a considerable investment, there are many things to be aware before choosing a school...

Do Your Research!

All makeup schools are not created equal. The truth is, fraud and misrepresentation do exist. There are stories all over the internet about fly by night schools. These schools will put up a professional looking website and basically tell you anything you want to hear. Once you fall for the fake pictures, testimonials and credentials they'll ask for some money to reserve your seat in class. After "reserving your seat" you'll soon discover there is no class, the phone number is disconnected and somehow the website vanished into thin air!

Please don't fall victim to these horrible scams. Do your research before handing any money over to anyone. In order to assist you, we compiled a few resources that can provide you useful information:

Visit Themakeupartist.com
- Click Q & A in the menu to see reported School Scams,

Student-School Agreement & more info about choosing the right school.

Do a Google search for:
- (Makeup school name) + scam
- Look for Reviews and opinions

Check with:
- BetterBusinessBureau.com
- RipOffReport.com

Inquire if the school is operating legally in the state they're in: Contact the State Board of Education and give them the school's name. You can also visit the National Association of State Boards of Education at nasbe.org for more info.

If possible try to visit the school in person. Do the pictures match the website? Is it clean and well kept? What is the overall vibe you get?

The Next Step

If a school checks out as far as scams go, the next step is to find out about the quality of the education they provide. We encourage you to ask the following questions. You may be able to find the answers on the school's website. If not, the school's admissions director should be able to assistance you.

- Is the curriculum general or does it specialize in one specific area?
- Do you provide "safe beauty" or "makeup hygiene" training?
- How much time is actually spent on reading from a text book vs. hands on practice?
- What credentials/experience does my instructor have? Can I see their published work?

- Will I receive a diploma/certificate when I complete the course?
- Can I receive pro artist discounts on makeup and supplies with my diploma/cert?

- Does the cost of the class include a kit to practice with?
- Are there any materials that the cost of the course does not cover?
- Will I be building a portfolio? Will the school provide a professional photographer?
- Does the school provide models to practice on or will I be required to bring in my own?
- Does the course focus on career guidance, business training & marketing?
- Does the school offer apprenticeship, intern programs or job placement assistance?
- Is student financing available?

While this research process can be time consuming, it can definitely save you money and headaches down the road. The most important thing to remember is never hand over any money until you are 100% sure about a school's professional credibility.

Helpful Resources

To find a directory of credible makeup schools around the world visit Makeupmag.com/schools & HMArtistsnetwork.com.

13 Alternative Learning Tools & Training Resources

When time, money or location makes it difficult to attend a makeup school, you do have alternative options. Although most options do not award you with a diploma/certificate, the knowledge you'll acquire is what ultimately counts. Alternative options include:

- Video Tutorials
- Books
- Home Study courses
- One on one coaching
- Workshops
- Assist a makeup artist

Tip: You'll need a face to practice so you can use your own or ask family/friends to volunteer. Paper makeup charts and makeup mannequins are also great to practice on. You can find makeup charts at the following retailers:

- thefacechart.com
- amazon.com
- mudshop.com
- makeupart.net
- robertjonesbeauty.com.

A quick online search of "how to fill out makeup chart" will provide further instructions. Makeup mannequins are another alternative. They are reusable and come in a variety of skin tones. You can find them at makeupart.net.

Video Tutorials

Watching video tutorials is one of the best and affordable ways to learn. Videos help expand your knowledge as it provides an opportunity to see people with different complexions, skin tones, face shapes and eye shapes apply makeup. It's a great way to learn about color selection and placement techniques based on persons' unique features/attributes.

But finding the best videos can be a time consuming process. So to help you out we sifted through thousands to create 'The Little Black Book of Celebrity Makeup Artists'. This resource guide provides you with the names and YouTube channels of world renowned A-list celebrity makeup artists as well as professional makeup brands and makeup "gurus". You'll learn firsthand from the masters about beauty makeup application and so much more.

In addition to YouTube, you can find video tutorials on almost every cosmetic brand's website. Cosmetic companies use professional makeup artists to demonstrate their products, so it's another great way to learn from the pros.

Books and DVDs

Amazon.com is an excellent source for books & DVD's that cover everything from beauty makeup, beyond beauty makeup as well as career related topics.

Popular titles include:

Books on Beauty makeup application

- Make-Up Designory's Beauty Make-Up by Yvonne Hawker
- Bobbi Brown Makeup Manual: For Everyone from Beginner to Pro by Bobbi Brown
- Makeup The Ultimate Guide by Rae Morris
- Make-up Masterclass: Beauty Bible of Professional Techniques and Wearable Looks by Jemma Kidd
- Makeup Your Mind: Express Yourself by Francois Nars

Books on Beyond Beauty makeup application

- Make-up Designory Character Makeup by Paul Thompson and Gil Romero
- Special Makeup Effects for Stage and Screen: Making and Applying Prosthetics by Todd Drebreceni

Home Study Courses

If you are unable to travel or dedicate the time needed for traditional on-site learning, you may consider a home study course. These courses are an excellent option is you would like to earn a certificate/diploma. Much like makeup schools, courses can vary considerably. Some focus on just makeup application. Others teach you skills specific to your career choice as well as makeup application. Before you commit to a home study course its best to know what you are paying for.

Ask the following questions:

- Will I receive a diploma or certificate when I complete the course?
- How many assignments and quizzes are required to complete the course?
- How much time is given to complete each assignment and quiz?

Please refer to the last section 'How to Choose a Makeup School' for more important questions to ask and how to find out if a home study course is a scam.

Popular home study courses found online are:

- Distant Learning Course - themakeoverstudio.com
- E Pro Image Courses -eproimagecourses.com

- Erin Shaw Online- erinshawmakeupacademy.com.au
- Hex Makeup Online -hexmakeupartist.com
- NOMA USA Online- nomausa.com
- QC Makeup Academy -qcmakeupacademy.com
- Robert Jones Online- robertjonesbeautyacademy.com
- RPM Online Courses -makeuponlinetraining.com
- Special Effects Training- dicksmithmake-up.com

One on One Coaching

One on one coaching enables you hire a makeup artist for career guidance based on your personal situation. A great advantage of this type of training is being able to ask questions and advice. Find a mentor at:

- Makeuplessons.com
- Makeupmentors.com
- Hmartistsnetwork.com/one-on-one-apprenticing

Workshops

Workshops are an excellent way to attend an instructor led class without the commitment of a makeup school. The length of a workshop varies considerably. Some last a few hours, while others may take a few days. Many workshops are offered at trade shows annually and are often taught by world renowned makeup artists. Popular trade shows include:

- International Beauty Show (IBS)
- International Makeup Artist Trade Show (IMATS)
- The Makeup Show

Popular workshops found online include:

- The Powder Group's Makeup 101 Workshop - thepowdergroup.com

- Rain Makeup Academy Beginners Artistry Workshop - rainmakeupacademy.com

- Mario Dedivanovic Workshops- blog.makeupbymario.com

- Jemma Kidd Academy's Introduction to Professional Make-up Artistry Workshop and Principles of Professional Make-up Artistry Workshop - academy.jemmakidd.com

- Face Stockholm's Makeup Artist Boot Camp Workshop and Professional Makeup Artist Workshop - facestockholm.com

- Candace Corey's The Makeup Artist Workshop - candacecorey.com

- Koloring with Kolors Makeup Workshop - kellikolors.com

- Find a list of upcoming workshops on the Hair & Makeup Artist Network - hmartistsnetwork.com

Assist an Artist

Assisting a professional makeup artist provides you with an opportunity to learn from someone with years of experience. Assistants get a chance to watch, listen and study a pro and build connections in the process. Contact an artist directly and let them know you're interested in learn by becoming their assistance.

Find a pro in your area by visiting:

- Hmartistsnetwork.com
- Makeup talent agencies
- Modelmayhem.com
- Yelp.com

14 The Little Black Book of Celebrity Makeup Artists

When it comes to developing your makeup skills, learning from experts and experienced professionals is always the best option but is often very expensive. Fortunately for you it's easy to access world class training taught by A-list celebrity makeup artists & the best part is it doesn't cost a penny!

Thanks to social sharing sites like Youtube.com, many celebrity makeup artists have created "virtual classrooms" to share their tips, tricks and expertise. You can learn all you nccd to know about all styles of beauty makeup at your own pace and from the comfort of your own home.

In addition to celebrity makeup artists you will also find a list of channels for professional makeup brands and makeup "gurus" that offer instructional tutorials on beauty and beyond beauty makeup.

We highly recommend you watch as many different makeup artists and videos as possible. No two makeup artists are exactly alike and you'll learn there are many ways to achieve the same results. Watch, listen and learn. Then apply what you've learned by practicing on yourself, a friend, paper face chart or a makeup mannequin.

Makeup charts are available at these online retailers:

- thefacechart.com
- amazon.com
- shopmud.com
- makeupart.net
- robertjonesbeauty.com

A quick online search of "how to fill out makeup chart" will provide further instructions. Makeup mannequins come in a variety of skin tones and are available at makeupart.net.

YouTube Tip

Most channels are organized by video playlists. You can save any existing playlist or customize your own. For example, you can create a playlist for each style of beauty makeup (clean beauty, basic beauty, fashion, glamour, bridal/special occasion & high fashion). You can also create categories for specific techniques or perhaps for looks that you like.

To get started, access each channel directly on Youtube.com.

Celebrity Makeup Artist Channels

Lisa Eldridge
Channel name: lisaeldrigedotcom & CHANEL

Lisa Eldridge is a professional A-list celebrity and editorial makeup artist. Her work has graced the cover of Vogue, Elle and the red carpet so much more. She's also a global beauty ambassador for Chanel. Her channel, lisaeldridgedotcom guides you through basic and advanced beauty makeup techniques. You can also find makeup tutorials by Lisa on channel CHANEL.

Charlotte Tilbury
Channel name: Charlotte Tilbury and NETAPORTER

Charlotte Tilbury is a high fashion celebrity makeup artist. She responsible for many of the looks we see on Kristen Stewart, Kate Moss, Victoria Secret super models, Mercedes Benz Fashion Week shows and covers of international fashion magazines.

Eve Pearl
Channel name: evepearl

Learn basic and advanced beauty makeup from a 5 time Grammy award winning makeup artist. Eve Pearl shares her tips and tricks she has acquired from18 years of experience. Eve Pearl is also the author of Plastic Surgery without the Surgery (available on amazon.com).

Samantha Chapman
Channel name: Pixiwoo

Samantha Chapman is an accomplished celebrity makeup artist with more than a decade of experience working in the fashion, music and TV industry.   Samantha shares her beauty makeup expertise along with her sister Nic on her channel Pixiwoo.

Lori Taylor
Channel name: giovannismash

 Lori Taylor is the lead makeup artist for Smashbox Cosmetics. Her modern and fresh approach to beauty leaves models and celebrities glowing.

Anastasia Soare
Channel name: AnastasiaBeverlyHill

Anatastasia Soare is known as the definitive brow expert. Her roaster of celebrity clientele includes the likes of Oprah, Madonna and Jennifer Lopez to name a few. Her channel AnastasiaBeverlyHill will show you how to achieve perfect brows every time and much more.

Rae Morris
Channel name: raemorrismakeup

Rae Morris is the go to makeup artist for A-listers like Cyndi Lauper, Cate Blanchette and many others. Learn her unique approach to makeup for women of all ages on her channel raemorrismakeup. Rae Morris is also the author of Makeup: The Ultimate Guide, Timeless Makeup & Beautiful Eyes: The Eye Makeup Guide (available on amazon.com).

Scott Barnes
Channel name: scottbarnestv

Learn from the man who gave JLO her famous glow. Scott Barnes' other famous clients include Kim Kardashian, Celine Dion, Christina Aguilera and a host of other A-list celebrities. Scott Barnes is also the author of About Face and Face to Face: Amazing New Looks and Inspiration from the Top Celebrity Makeup Artist (available on amazon.com).

Mally Roncal
Channel name: mallytvproductions

 Mally Roncal is a celebrity makeup artist and founder of Mally Beauty cosmetics. One of her biggest celebrity clients is Beyonce. You find her personality is just as beautiful as her makeup. Visit Mally on her channel mallytvproductions.

Robert Jones
Channel name: robertjonesbeauty

Robert Jones is an international makeup artist. His extensive list of celebrity clientele includes Cindy Crawford, Selena Gomez, Sheryl Crow, Leeann Rimes and so many more. Visit Robert on his channel robertjonesbeauty.

Gucci Westman
Channel name: revlon

Meet world renowned makeup and Revlon's creative director Gucci Westman. Her celebrity clientele includes Drew Barrymore, Jennifer Aniston, Gwyneth Paltrow, and Natalie Portman. Learn Gucci's wearable approach to beauty makeup on channel revlon.

Bobbi Brown
Channel name: bobbibrown

The founder of Bobbi Brown cosmetics walks you through her natural approach to celebrity beauty. She is also the author of Bobbi Brown Makeup Manual: For Everyone from Beginner to Pro (available on amazon.com).

Pat McGrath
Channel name: CoverGirl & dolcegabbanachannel

Path McGrath is the artistic director for Cover Girl and Dolce & Gabanna makeup. Her work has graced the covers of high fashion magazines and supermodels during Fashion Week. She can be found on channel CoverGirl and dolcegabbanachannel.

Sarah Uslan
Channel name: sarahuslan

Sarah Uslan is a highly sought out celebrity makeup artist. Her clients include Rose McGowan, Amy Poehler and many others. Learn easy techniques that deliver red carpet results on her channel sarahuslan.

Carlene K
Channel name: carlenekmakeup

Carlene K works with an extensive list of celebrities including Nicole Scherzinger, Britney Spears, Ericka Jayne and many others. She was also the official artist for the Pussycat Dolls. Learn her unique approach to beauty makeup on her channel carlenekmakeup.

Kevin James Bennett
Channel name: Kevin James Bennett

Kevin James Bennett is a multi Emmy award winning makeup artist. This world class educator brings 25 years of expertise to his channel Kevin James Bennett.

Kabuki
Channel name: KabukimagicNYC & myfacecosmetics

Kabuki is a world renowned celebrity makeup artist. He was the official makeup artist for Sarah Jessica Parker for Sex and the City. He also works with superstars like Katy Perry and Rhianna. Learn from Kabuki on his channel KabukimagicNYC and myfacecosmetics.

Wendy Rowe
Channel name: Burberry

Wendy Rowe is the artistic beauty consultant for Burberry cosmetics. Her work is featured in international magazines like Harper's Bazaar and Italian Vogue. She also designs the makeup looks for many runway shows during New York Fashion Week. She can be found on channel Burberry.

Sonia Kashuk
Channel name: SoniaKashukInc

Sonia Kashuk's clients include Vogue, Harper's Bazaar, Allure, Elle and Glamour to name a few. She has worked with the likes of Cindy Crawford and is also the creator of the cosmetic brand Sonia Kashuk. Meet Sonia on her channel SoniaKashukInc.

Makeup Brands Official Channels

- Benefit Cosmetics
- Illamasqua
- MACcosmetics
- Mufepro (Makeup Forever)
- Sephora
- SmashboxCosmetics
- Stilavideo
- Makeupdesignory
- NARS Media
- UrbanDecay YT

Beauty Makeup Guru Channels

- Ateliermaquillage
- Beatfacehoney

- Beautyartstudio
- Blushbeautytutor
- Deepaberar
- Destiny Godley
- Givegoodface
- Guatemalanhotmama1
- Gossmakeupartist
- Hagai Avdar
- Jhmemoires
- Kandeejohnson
- Klairedelysart
- Look TV
- Lipshock
- MakeupGeekTV
- MakeupTalk
- Maria Maslarski
- Mickiyagi Hirschmann
- MsCreativeDiva
- Msroshposh
- Myeyeshadowisodd
- Naeemkhanmakeup
- Nikkietutorials
- Petjachannel
- Petrilude
- Prettylilmzgrace
- Priscilla Ono
- Qazimediagroup
- Sculptbeautytv
- Sokolum79
- Thefancyfaced
- TheFolaron
- Tymetheinfamous
- Weedaa11
- ZunetaBeauty

Beyond Beauty Makeup Guru Channels

- Anaarthur81
- Brickintheyark
- Dope2111
- FabaTV
- Fumsmusings
- Goldiestarling
- Jinny Genevieve Houle
- Petrilude
- Stan Winston School

Chapter 4
Exploring Career Options

In This Chapter:

- Weighing Your Options
- What is a Freelance Makeup Artist?
- Exploring a Career in Cosmetic Sales
- Exploring a Career in Personal Beauty Service
- Exploring a Career in Media Production

15 Weighing Your Options

Professional makeup artistry is essentially comprised of three industries which are:

- Cosmetic retail sales
- Personal beauty service
- Media production

In this chapter, we'll introduce you to the various career options that each industry has to offer. As you explore your options, please be honest with yourself about your passion, current lifestyle & how much change you are open to. Ask yourself:

- Are you looking for steady employment or a chance to run your own business and be your own boss?
- Which industries exist where you live?
- If the industries don't exist, are you willing to move to where they are?

These questions will hopefully help you clarify what you're willing/not willing to do to pursue a new career. The beautiful thing about makeup artistry is that there are many options that don't require a drastic change and you don't have to live in a big city, to build a career you can be proud of. After exploring your career options, refer to Chapters 5-7 to learn what it takes to get started.

16   What Is A Freelance Makeup Artist?

In makeup artistry, freelance refers to a makeup artist who is self-employed. Being self-employed means that you're a business owner. It also means that you are your own employee.

A freelancer (or independent contractor) generally works with one client at a time with no long term commitment. In other words, once you complete the job (laid out in a written agreement/contract) you're no longer tied to your client.

As a business owner a freelancer is responsible for:

- Keeping track of business expenses & money coming in
- File and pay personal & business income taxes
- Obtain your own health insurance & other benefits
- Obtain makeup artist liability insurance

In addition to duties of running a managing a business, a freelancer is also in charge of finding work through marketing and self-promotion. To be successful at finding work it's imperative that a freelancer acquires sales skills as well as customer service skills.

The Difference between Self-Employment & Employment

Being an employee and being self-employed are as different as night and day. An employee is committed to a company that compensates them for their time/performance with a wage or salary. They typically have a job title and specified duties assigned by a supervisor. Another major difference is that your employer is responsible for withholding your personal income tax from your earnings. And finally, most employers often provide health insurance & retirement benefits on your behalf.

To learn more about freelancing, sales and customer service skills we've gathered a list of resources and learning tools:

The U.S. Small Business Administration

The SBA provides information and links on how to set up and run your business. They also provide articles, news and mentor programs. Visit sba.gov for more information.

Jan Zobel

Jan Zobel is a tax preparer with over 20 years of experience, wrote Minding Her Own Business, The Self-Employment Woman's Guide to Taxes and Record Keeping with the newbie in mind. This book provides an insightful and comprehensive look at the basics of starting & running a business. Purchase your copy today on amazon.com.

Legal Zoom

Let Legal Zoom take care of all the hassle of preparing and filing legal documents to start your business. They also have licensed attorney available to give you legal advice. Visit legalzoom.com for more info.

Freelancers Union

Freelancers Union supports and protects the interest of freelancers. In addition to giving freelancer's a political voice they also provide health, dental, disability, life and retirement insurance. Visit freelancersunion.com

i Makeup Matters

Learn about the risks associated with being a makeup artist & how to protect yourself with public liability insurance. Visit imakeupmatters.com for more information.

Books on building Customer Service skills

Be Our Guest, Perfecting the Art of Customer Service by The Disney Institute and Theodore Kinni (revised and updated edition)

Customer Satisfaction is Worthless, Customer Loyalty is Priceless: How to Make Them Love You, Keep You Coming Back, and Tell Everyone They Know by Jeffrey H. Gitomer

Books on building Sales skills

How to Master the Art of Selling by Tom Hopkins

17   Exploring a Career in Cosmetic Retail Sales

Type of makeup applied in Cosmetic Retail Sales:

- Beauty

Type of Beauty makeup styles:

- Clean beauty
- Basic beauty
- Fashion
- Glamour
- Bridal/Special Occasion

As a makeup artist working sales, your objective is to help customers find suitable makeup for their personal use. A part of the sales process involves one on one consultation to determine the customers' need. It also involves demonstrating makeup application and educating the customer about the benefits of the products. Makeup artists working in this industry are commonly referred to as 'product consultants' or 'beauty advisors'.

Occasionally, you will have customers in need of makeup for special occasions like weddings (brides/bridal party), prom, anniversaries, etc. In those cases the person may schedule a time to see you and have their makeup done for the actual event. In exchange for the makeup application, they will purchase all or some of the makeup you used on them.

Career paths within Cosmetic Retail Sales include:

- Freestanding stores
- Department store counters
- Direct-sales organizations

Freestanding Stores & Department Store Counters

Freestanding stores & department store counters generally hire makeup artists as employees for part time to full time positions (although its becoming more common for stores/counters to hire freelancers). You can expect to earn an hourly wage or commission based on your sales performance. Other duties besides consultation/makeup application may include ringing up sales, taking inventory, keeping the sales area clean, participating in promotional events & more.

Direct Sales Organizations

Direct Sales Organizations like Avon & Mary Kay allow makeup artists to get started with their own home based business with a small investment. As a direct sales "beauty consultant" you can set your own work schedule and reach customers via in-person, online and through mobile devices. In this area of cosmetic retail sales you are considered self-employed and earn a percentage on each sale you make. Working as your own boss includes responsibilities such as marketing and networking to find customers, keeping track of orders/shipments/deliveries, handling finances and organizing your schedule.

Other direct sales companies besides Avon and Mary Kay include: Arbonne, Affordable Minerals Makeup, Ava Anderson, Beauti Control, Jafra, FM Cosmetics and Motives Cosmetics (Market America).

Careers in Cosmetic Retail Sales Can Lead to More Opportunities

Many makeup artists begin their professional careers in Cosmetic Retail Sales and use it as a stepping stone to advance to the Personal

Beauty Service and/or Media Production industry. They utilize their time in sales to gain experience in customer service/business, become knowledgeable about cosmetics, practice applying makeup on a variety of people and most importantly network. Another valuable benefit is the employee discount many cosmetic companies offer, which allows you to build a kit at a fraction of the price.

Working for cosmetic company can lead also lead to work in media productions (typically fashion related). Cosmetic companies like M.A.C. Cosmetics offer opportunities for their employees to become part of a pro team. Typically to be accepted in a pro team, you'll need experience in cosmetic retail sales, demonstrate professionalism & artistic talent. As a member of a pro team, you travel and participate in media productions that range from editorial photo shoots to live events. MAC is actually renowned for doing makeup for the biggest fashion event in the world - Mercedes Benz Fashion Week. Recently, M.A.C. teamed up with Milk Studios in N.Y.C. to create their own fashion event called Made Fashion Week.

To learn more about Cosmetic Retail Sales, the beauty industry and/or direct sales we recommend the following books:

- The Beauty Industry by Paula Black

- Estee Lauder: Doyenne of Beauty (Titans of Fortune) by Daniel Elef

- Color Stories - Behind the Scenes of America's Billion-Dollar Beauty Industry by Mary Lisa Gavenas

- Avon Building the World's Premier Company for Women by Laura Klepacki

- Mary Kay Ash: Queen of Sales (Titans of Fortune) by Daniel Elef

18   Exploring a Career in Personal Beauty Service

Type of makeup applied in Personal Beauty Service:

- Beauty

Type of makeup styles:

- Clean beauty
- Basic beauty
- Fashion
- Glamour
- Bridal/Special Occasion

Personal Beauty Service makeup artists are sought out for brides, bridal parties and for other meaningful events like anniversaries, prom & graduations. This kind of makeup artist is often referred to as bridal or event makeup artist.

The process of providing makeup services includes makeup trials/consultations. During a trial/consultation you ask questions to determine a person's skin type, their use of cosmetics and the look they would like to achieve. A full makeup application is also included in trial/consultation.

While it is possible to find employment, the majority of makeup artists in this industry are self-employed. When working as your own boss you are responsible for marketing and networking to find clients, keeping track of finances and appointments.

Working with others in the industry

An important thing to keep in mind is that hairstylists also play an active role in the personal beauty service industry. Therefore, it's not uncommon for a makeup artist to have to work alongside a hairstylist if they are both working for the same client/event.

Career paths within Personal Beauty Service include:

- Salons
- Spas
- Mobile Service

Salons & Spas

Salons and spas offer a makeup artist a stationary location to work from. They also provide a great opportunity to build a clientele who prefer a "one stop shop" for their beauty needs (makeup, hair, nails, facials, waxing, etc.) As an employee at these establishments, you can expect to earn an hourly wage or commission. Those who are self-employed earn income from walk-ins and clientele they find themselves (often by word of mouth referrals). Typically, you pay the salon/spa a percentage of your earnings or a monthly rental fee for a work station/booth. The amount you can charge your clientele for your services greatly depends on the salon/spa's policies.

Mobile Service

A Mobile Service or on-location makeup artist travels to various clients and applies makeup either at their home or requested location (example: hotel room where the bride is getting ready or a private room where reception is taking place). This type of makeup artist is a self-employed freelancer and finds clients through marketing efforts and word of mouth referrals.

Work hours can vary greatly for a mobile makeup artist. While it's not a typical 9-5 job, is it possible to earn a full day's pay within a few hours. The rates/price you charge can be set and negotiated at your discretion. When establishing your rates/prices, important factors to consider are travel expenses (gas/mileage), the value of your makeup kit, and the value of your time if you are asked to stay at the event to touch up your client's makeup (powder, lipstick, etc).

To learn more about the Personal Beauty Service and the bridal industry we recommend the following books:

Salon & Spa

- To Rent or Not to Rent by Judiffier Pearson
- Minding Your Own Business: What Every Salon Owner, Booth Renter and Independent Contractor Should Know by Judiffier Pearson

Mobile Service

Mobile Cosmetic Business by Tim Roncevich and Steven Primm

Bridal industry

One Perfect Day: The Selling of the American Wedding by Rebecca Mead

19 Exploring a Career in Media Production

Type of makeup applied in Media Production:

- Beauty
- Makeup artists interested in television, movies and theater also need to be skilled in applying Beyond Beauty makeup.*

Type of Beauty makeup styles:

- Clean beauty
- Basic beauty
- Fashion
- Glamour
- Bridal/Special Occasion
- High Fashion

*Type of Beyond Beauty makeup styles:

- Character
- Special Effects

Media production is by far the most complex career path in makeup artistry. It's a very large industry that offers an abundance of choices. Because the internet makes it possible to distribute media at a very low cost, there's been a rapid growth of production companies worldwide.

Media production companies specialize in one or more of the following:

- Commercial photography
- Video production
- Television production
- Movie production

- Theater/stage production
- Live Event production

The Role of a Media Makeup Artist

Working on a production involves collaborating with a team of people to design a specific look or character. Depending on the type of production your involved in, you could work closely with:

- Photographers/directors
- Art or creative directors
- Production designer
- Hair stylists
- Other makeup artists
- Makeup Teams
- Wardrobe designers/stylists
- Lighting technicians
- Camera technicians
- Event coordinators

The type of production will also determine what type of "talent" you'll apply makeup on - actors, models, celebrities, singers/entertainers, politicians, athletes, public figures, etc. are considered the "talent". Work environments include but are not limited to dressing rooms, green rooms, studios, sets, trailers, backstage, or outdoors in a variety of weather conditions.

There are two titles, one of which a makeup artist is appointed on a production. The first is known as a "key makeup artist" who is in charge of managing the makeup department. As the key you are responsible for overseeing supplies, accounting for weather conditions (wind, temperature and humidity extremes) as well as the electrical supply for artificial lighting, fans, etc, when working outdoors. Sometimes when a production such a movie involves special effects/prosthetics there will be a separate "Special FX makeup artist" that the key consults with. The other title is known as an "assistant". The assistant is typically hired by the key and is given duties to perform such as- cleaning dirty makeup brushes, keeping the makeup area organized and prepping the talent(s) for the makeup application and sometimes apply makeup.

The majority makeup artists in media are freelancers & act as their own managers unless they find representation through an agency, union or cosmetic company pro team. Managing yourself means marketing your portfolio/services to find work, negotiating pay/work terms with production co., sending invoices/billing for your services and managing your finances. You'll also be responsible for obtaining the appropriate license(s) & filing taxes.

One of the most important elements of working on any production is building professional relationships with the production co., talent, staff as well as other stylists (hair, wardrobe and even other makeup artists). These connections are important as they can lead to more work opportunities. Often if the talent likes working with the makeup artist, they will request or personally hire them for promotional work and/or other projects. For example, let's say a production co. hired you to apply makeup on an actress. If you make a good impression, that actress may want to continue to work with you and hire you for promotional work (photo shoots, guest appearances meet and greets, magazine covers, red carpet events, interviews, galas, premiers, etc).

A Closer Look at Media Production Companies

Commercial Photography Production Companies

Commercial photographers work with still capture cameras that are either digital or use film to produce "print" and "digital" visual media. "Print" refers to an image being printed on material such as paper. "Digital" implies an image in electronic form (on a website for example).

Working with a photographer doesn't always mean you'll be in a studio. Because the needs of each client are different, photographers

can find themselves shooting outdoors or in unpredictable settings.
Some assignments may require you to travel.

While some photographers are active in the creative direction of a
shoot, others rely on an Art Director to guide them. It's the Art
Directors responsibility to overlook the visual impact of a photo.
This includes making sure the clothes, hair, makeup, setting and
mood are in line with what the client wants.

Makeup artists work in the following areas of photography:

- Commercial
- Fashion
- Editorial
- Portfolio

What is Commercial photography?

While all photographers in media production are known as
"commercial photographers", not all photographers take pictures in
this commercial style sense. In commercial style photography
businesses/corporations hire photographers to capture images that
showcase the company/brand or to highlight a product/service they
provide. Commercial images are used for promotional and
advertising purposes – campaigns, billboards, brochures, websites,
catalogues, magazines and other publications. Typically,
"commercial style" work is known to pay the most out of all types of
photography assignments.

What is Editorial photography?

Publications (newspaper/magazines) hire photographers to capture
images that help support a story - known as an editorial. Not to be
confused with an advertisement, an editorial basically provides a
reader with entertaining or informative content. It's important to
recognize that there are many different types of publications that

range from women's interest to men's interest and everything in between. Some editorial photographers focus on certain styles of editorial, for example fashion for Vogue magazine. The internet has provided an opportunity for publications to avoid the high costs of printing by going digital. Because of this, there are an ever-growing number of new publications every year which makes for the high demand of editorial photographers as well as makeup artists.

What is Fashion photography?

Fashion photography is one the most recognized form of commercial photography. A fashion photographer specializes in photographing clothes, shoes and accessories. Fashion images can be used for catalogues, websites, ad campaigns, magazine editorials and marketing material. There are several of styles and techniques in commercial fashion photography. For example, images for printed catalogues and online stores attempt to show the details of the clothing. While editorial shots, attempt to present clothes in more unusual and creative ways. Generally "high fashion" or "haute couture" photographers are based out of the fashion capitals of the world – New York, London, Paris, and Milan. More recently, Miami, Los Angeles, Hong Kong, Sydney and Mumbai have become recognized as 'fashion capitals'.

What is Portfolio photography?

Models, actors, musicians and other types of talent seek portfolio photographers to take head shots and concept or creative portraits for their professional portfolios. Head shots intend to show the subject in a very natural way from the shoulders up. Concept/creative portraits attempt to show a more diverse side of the person. Wardrobe, makeup, hair, lighting and setting all play an important role in concept photography.

To learn more about commercial photography media productions, we recommend the following learning tools:

- Fashion Photography Exposed DVD by Melissa Rodwell, available on *fashionphotography.com*

- Advertising Photography: A Straightforward Guide to a Complex Industry by Lou Lesko

- The Art and Business of Photography by Susan Carr

- Fashion Photography: A Complete Guide to the Tools & Tricks of the Trade by Bruce Smith

- Fashion Photography 101 by Lara Jade

Video Production Companies

You'll find that many commercial photographers also shoot video. Working in this medium makes them a videographer. Video production use motion capture cameras to produce content intended for broadcast or non-broadcast purposes. Broadcast refers to video that will be seen via television. Non-broadcast also known as "new media" refers to video used for web distribution (on a website or a video sharing platform like YouTube).

A video production company can have clients that range from small local business to international corporations in need of:

- Advertising (commercials)
- Promotion & Marketing
- Music
- Corporate
- Training/Tutorials
- Event coverage

On behalf of their clients a video production co. handles the concept development, writing the script, directing, casting and more. The needs of the clients determine if a video will be shot in studio, on location or in a combination of places.

To learn more about video media production, we recommend the following books.

- The Business of Media Distribution: Monetizing Film, TV & Video Content in an Online World by Jeff Ulin

- The 30-Second Storyteller: The Art and Business of Directing Commercials by Thomas Richter

- TV Commercials: How to Make Them or How Big is the Boat? by Ivan Cury

- Making Music Videos: Everything you Need to Know from the Best in the Business by Laura M Schwartz

- Experiencing Music Video: Aesthetics and Cultural Context by Carol Vernallis

TV & Movie Production Companies

Television and movie production companies use motion capture cameras to produce entertaining, enlightening and/or educational content. TV programs are broadcasted either through a network, cable, satellite or on-demand web streaming. Movies are generally showcased at film festivals then distributed through theaters for public viewing. (The term "movie" is interchangeable with motion picture, cinema and film - even if the movie is produced in a digital format).

There are essentially four key players for a TV or movie production. They are the writer, director, the DP (director of photography aka cinematographer) and producer(s). The writer develops a story or script, the director oversees the actors in relation to the script, the DP is responsible for making artistic & technical decisions related to the cameras and the image & finally the producer obtains financing for the production. It's common for one person to handle one or more of these roles especially on low budget and/or independent projects.

TV and movie production companies generally fall under 2 categories. The first is either owned or under contract with a network/studio system – based in Los Angeles, California- and includes major studios, entertainment companies, motion picture companies or media conglomerates. The other type work mostly or completely outside of a studio system are known as independents or "indie". Independent productions that utilize the studio systems for some support are known as 'mainstream independents'. Those who work entirely outside a studio system are known as "completely independent'.

Independent productions grew out of the advancement of digital motion capture cameras and editing software. This new media has allowed people to produce and broadcast/distribute content at lower costs (thanks to the internet) and with more creative control than they could with traditional networks and studio systems. The amount of independent productions throughout US and internationally are continuing to increase exponentially.

The various types of TV production genres include: Competition, Dramas, Family, Game, Lifestyle, Mystery, News, Reality, Scientific, Shopping, Sitcoms, Soaps, Talent & Talk

Movie fall into two categories:

- Short films (runs around 40 minutes including credits)
- Feature films (exceeds 40 minutes)

Movie genres include: Action, Children's, Comedy, Crime, Documentary, Drama, Family, Horror, Mystery, Romance, Science Fiction & Thriller/Suspense.

To learn more about TV and movie productions we recommend the following books:

- Technical Film and TV for Nontechnical People by Drew

Campbell

- Hollywood 101: The Film Industry by Frederick Levy

- How Movies Work by Bruce F. Kawin

- The Business of Television by Howard J. Blumenthal

- Independent Feature Film Production: A Complete Guide from Concept Through Distribution by Gregory Goodell

- Cinema of Outsiders: The Rise of American Independent Film by Emanuel Levy

Other books related to TV & Movie Production:

- The Story of Hollywood: An Illustrated History by Gregory Paul Williams
- The Glamour Factor: Inside Hollywood's Big Studio System by Ronald L. Davis
- Soap Opera Acting: The Ins and Out of Daytime Drama by Bonnie Forward
- Reality TV: An Insider's Guide to Today's Hottest Market by Troy DeVolld
- Starstruck: The Business of Celebrities by Elizabeth Currid-Halkett

Theater/Stage Production Companies

Theater and stage is a type of media production that is performed in front of a live audience. In this medium, you work with a production company that either resides or rents a venue to perform at. There are also touring companies that travel and perform in different cities.

Much like a TV or movie production, there are 3 key players: writer (playwright), director and producer(s). Another important person is known as the stage manager. This person is responsible for supervising all aspects of a performance including casting, dress rehearsals, the stage, lighting, sound, etc.

Stage productions are generally divided into 3 categories which include
dance, performance & pageant.

Cirque du Soleil is an example of a theater production that falls into more than one category– it's a hybrid of dramatic mix of circus arts and street entertainment.

To learn more about theater and stage productions, we recommend the following books:

- Technical Theater for Non-Technical People by Drew Campbell

- Theatrical Design and Production: An Introduction to Scene Design and Construction, Lighting, Sound, Costume, and Makeup by J. Michael Gillette

- The Back Stage Guide to Stage Management, 3rd Edition: Traditional and New Methods for Running a Show from First Rehearsal to Last Performance by Thomas A. Kelly

- Producing Beauty Pageants: A Director's Guide by Anna Stanley

Live Event Production Companies

The most notable live event associated with makeup artists are fashion industry events - better known as fashion runway shows. Fashion shows can be seen in many cities around the world and provide a platform for designers, brands and retailers to showcase the latest fashion.

The production of a show is carried out by a "show producer" or "show coordinator". It is their job to oversee all aspects of production on behalf of a fashion designer, brand or retailer. Many of those aspects include hiring a staff to assist with securing a venue, casting hair and makeup talent, casting models, lighting, sound-design, set design, rehearsals, and security for public safety.

Fashion shows are organized by the type of clothing first and then on the season.

Clothing type categories include: Bridal, Couture, Eco-Friendly, Mass Market, Menswear, Ready to Wear & Swimwear.

Seasonal fashion show categories include Spring/Summer, Pre-Fall, Fall/Winter & Resort.

The largest and most prestigious of all fashion shows are presented at an event called Fashion Week sponsored by Mercedes Benz. Originally, Mercedes Benz Fashion Week was held in the fashion capitals of the world – New York City, London, Milan and Paris. But since the first show in 1943, Fashion Week has expanded to 138 cities worldwide (and counting). The shows occur semi-annually and last approximately one week, hence the name "Fashion Week".

During this frenzy filled week, famous designers showcase their seasonal collections to a selective audience of media, luxury retailers, editors, stylists, celebrities, VIPs as well as fashion conscious people and "style experts". Although the shows are not open to the public, the internet has made virtual access possible to many shows through live broadcast on websites like Style.com.

There are many other fashion shows around the world that are not as exclusive as Mercedes Benz Fashion Week. While they still may use the term "Fashion Week", these shows provide a platform for less well known designers, mainstream brands and/or mass retailers. The clothes they feature are a lot more affordable and practical. Often the fashion being presented is inspired by high end designers you would see at Mercedes Benz Fashion Week. These types of shows are described as mass market or ready to wear. Many are open to the public.

To learn more about live event productions, we recommend the following books:

- How to Produce a Fashion Show from A to Z by Paula Taylor

- In Fashion, 2nd Edition by Elaine Stone

- New York Fashion Week: The Designers, the Models, the Fashions of the Bryant Park Era by Elia Mell

Additional Resources

Forums

Forums are a great opportunity to learn from other makeup artist's experiences, join the discussion and ask questions of your own. We highly recommend the following forums:

- Makeupandrelatedindustries.yuku.com
- Modelmayhem.com
- Hmartistsnetwork.com

Magazines

Magazines designed for makeup artists let you know what's new & happening in makeup artistry. Famous ones include:

- Makeup Artist Magazine (makeupmag.com)
- The Artisan (local706.org)
- Beauty Etc. (beautyetc.com)
- Face On (faceonmagazine.co.uk)

Trade Shows

Every year makeup artists from around the globe gather at trade shows to learn new skills, watch pro demos and discover new products. World renowned shows include:

- The Makeup Show
- International Makeup Artist Trade Show (IMATS)
- International Beauty Show (IBS)

Chapter 5
Getting Started in Cosmetic Retail Sales

In This Chapter:

- Building Essential Skills
- Building a Portfolio
- Jumpstarting Your Career

20   Building Essential Skills

If you decide you'd like to pursue a career in cosmetic retail sales, it's important to gain the right skills. Although there are courses available at makeup school for cosmetic sales, you may also consider alternative learning tools and training resources.

One of the best alternative training resources is working for a company that offers on the job training. Retail stores & makeup counters hire people with no experience and train them in makeup hygiene, beauty makeup application, customer service/sales skills and makeup brands. Others may require you to have at least basic sales skills but will train you in makeup hygiene, beauty makeup application, customer service and brands. Direct sales organizations typically provide training through instructional pamphlets and well as through online videos. The type of training you can expect is mainly sales/ promotion oriented. They do however offer how to videos and printed guides to assist you with makeup application.

The List of Essential Skills

Whatever training method you decide on its important to understand which skills you need to focus on building. Essential cosmetic retail sales skills fall into 4 categories:

- Safe Beauty
- Beauty Makeup
- HD Makeup
- Business

Safe Beauty Skills

The first skills you must acquire are disease control and prevention aka safe beauty skills. As we previously discussed, it may be required by law for you to obtain a cosmetology license. Please refer back to *Chapter 4 - Makeup Artist Licensing-* for more information and instructions.

Beauty Makeup Skills

Beauty makeup skills are the most essential and common skills used by makeup artists in cosmetic retail sales. Focus on learning the following types of Beauty styles:

- Clean beauty
- Basic beauty
- Fashion
- Glamour
- Bridal/Special Occasion

HD Skills

In addition to beauty makeup, we highly recommend HD makeup training. HD skills will serve you well as everyday women are now buying HD makeup for an "airbrushed look". Understanding the benefits of this makeup to relay to your customers and showing them how to properly apply it can translate to more sales.

Business Skills

Business skills are essential for professional growth. Most importantly, they will prepare you for providing quality professional service to your customers and clients. Business skills incorporate the following:

- Sales & Customer Service
- Self- Employed /Freelancing

Customer Service & Sales skills are essential in dealing with people and conveying the right message about your services. When applied correctly, these skills will earn you loyal lifetime clients and a strong referral base.

Self- Employed/Freelancer skills allow you run a business if your interested in a career as a freelancer in retail sales or direct sales. These skills include setting up a business, managing your finances, filing your taxes and obtaining personal/liability insurance.

21   Building a Portfolio

You do not necessarily need a "traditional" or "formal" portfolio to get started in cosmetic retail sales. Retail stores/makeup counters usually just ask you to fill out an application. You definitely won't need one in direct sales as your makeup skills have nothing do with becoming a representative.

 However, a portfolio can serve as a powerful sales tool. Showcasing your makeup skills can lead to more prospective customers wanting your help. They'll not only see you as sales person but as a true makeup artist.

The easiest way to start a portfolio is by using paper face charts. With makeup face charts you won't have to worry about finding models or photographers to take pictures of your work. They are fairly inexpensive and can be displayed nicely in a binder. Makeup charts also allow you to keep records of the products customer use.

A quick online search of 'how to fill out a face chart' will bring up numerous tutorials teaching you how to apply makeup on paper. Makeup face charts are available at the following online retailers.

- Thefacechart.com
- Mudshop.com (click on Books/Apparel)
- Amazon.com (search makeup face chart)
- Robertjonesbeauty.com (click on tools)
- Makeupart.net (click Shop – makeup, tools & accessories)

A new alternative to the paper face chart portfolio is a digital one. Apps like Face Chart Pro (available on facechartpro.com) allow you to create an array of looks and save them to your ipad, iphone or ipod touch (& eventually Androids). A great feature of this app is that you can easily adjust the skin tone from light to dark and every color in between. A fantastic benefit is that you don't even need real makeup so you can create face charts anytime, anywhere. It's also a great tool to create a personalized face chart for customer (listing the products you've used) and you can even email it to them.

If you'd interested in learning how to build a traditional/formal portfolio, you can find instructions in Chapters 6 and 7.

22   Jumpstarting Your Career

In this section we'll take guide you the general steps it takes to start working in retail stores/makeup counters and direct sales.

Retail Stores & Makeup Counters

Filling up an application is the first step towards working at a retail store /makeup counter. If you are called for an interview, be sure to prepare by researching information about the company. Looks at its history, mission statement and brands/products it carries. Knowing this information will show your interest in the company. You'll also want to be prepared to answer questions such as:

- Why do you want to work here?
- Where do you see yourself in 2 -5 years?

Interviewers ask these questions to find people that are a good fit for a company. It's equally important to know if a company is a good fit for you, so don't be afraid to ask questions yourself.

The hiring process is different for every company. Be prepared by doing some online research about the hiring process for the co. your interested in. You'll find many people share their experience on forums and offer 'what to do/what not to do" advice.

If you need assistance with your interviewing skills, there are many experts that offer advice and tips on YouTube (keyword search: interview skills).

We also recommend you read:

- How To Interview Like A Pro: Forty-Three Rules For Getting Your Next Job by JD Mary Greenwood

In addition to interviewing skills, we also recommend you learn how to create a skills-based resume. Whether or not you have work experience related to cosmetic retail sales, you can use a skills-based resume to highlight your strengths. Learn how to create one by searching "skills based resume".

Direct Sales Organizations

The process of becoming a direct sales rep. begins with filling out a registration form. These forms are usually available online. You basically need to provide general information about yourself and pay a onetime fee. Depending on the organization you choose, the fee typically ranges from $20 - $100.

What happens after filling out a registration form varies from org. to org. Some will connect you with a beauty consultant in your area who will act as your mentor/advisor. Others allow you set up your account to get started right away. Either way you can expect to receive a "welcome kit" or "starter kit" with the latest products and brochures to guide you.

Chapter 6

Getting Started in Personal Beauty Service

In This Chapter:

- Building Essential Skills
- Building a Portfolio
- Jumpstart Your Career

23   Building Essential Skills

If you decide you'd like to pursue a career in Personal Beauty
Service, it's crucial to gain the right skills. There are several options
when it comes to training. You might decide to attend a makeup
school or consider alterative learning tools/training resources.
Whichever route you choose, it's important to understand which
skills you need to build.

Essential skills fall into 4 categories:

- Safe Beauty
- Beauty Makeup
- Airbrush & HD
- Business

Safe Beauty Skills

The first skills you must acquire are disease control and prevention
aka safe beauty skills. As we previously discussed, it may be
required by law for you to obtain a cosmetology license. Please refer
back to *Chapter 4 - Makeup Artist Licensing-* for more information
and instructions.

Please note: If you're thinking about working in a salon/spa, you'll
most likely need a license (even if the state board doesn't require it).
However, there are makeup artists who can work without a license if
the salon/spa is willing to sponsor them. If you have an idea of a
salon/spa you want to work at be sure to ask them about this.

Beauty Makeup Skills

Beauty makeup skills are the most essential and common skills used
by personal beauty service makeup artists. Focus on learning the
following types of Beauty styles:

- Clean beauty
- Basic beauty
- Fashion
- Glamour
- Bridal/Special Occasion

Airbrush & HD Skills

Acquiring airbrush skills are essential as many brides request that service. HD skills allow you to apply makeup suited for high definition cameras. Since the majority of brides are now taking pictures in HD this is a very important skill to have.

Business Skills

Business skills are essential to for managing and growing your business. Most importantly, they will prepare you for providing quality professional service to your clients. Business skills incorporate the following:

- Bridal Service
- Self- Employed /Freelancing
- Sales & Customer Service

Bridal Service skills include conducting consultations/makeup trials, scheduling/managing your time as well as writing contracts.

Here are a few learning tools that can help you build your Bridal Service skills.

- The Bridal Beauty Mastery Course DVD, *caracosmetics.com*
- The Business of Bridal Business by KR Moehr, *amazon.com*
- How To Start A Home Based Makeup Artist Business by Deanna Nickel (Focus on Bridal), *amazon.com*

Self- Employed/Freelancer skills allow you run a business whether you decide to work in a salon/spa based or as a mobile makeup artist. These skills include setting up a business, managing your finances, filing your taxes and obtaining personal/liability insurance. Please refer back to Chapter 3 – What is a Freelance Makeup Artist – for freelancing learning tools and training resources

Customer Service & Sales skills are essential in dealing with people and conveying the right message about your services. When applied correctly, these skills will earn you loyal lifetime clients and a strong referral base. Please refer back to Chapter 3 – What is a Freelance Makeup Artist – for freelancing learning tools and training resources.

24   Building a Portfolio

Once you've had time to develop your skills to work as a personal beauty service makeup artist, you can begin focusing on building a portfolio. If you choose to acquire training through a makeup school, you'll want to find out if the school will assist you in building one. If they do not or if you choose not attend a school this section will get you started.

Getting Started

You can start to build an impressive bridal/special occasion portfolio with a little patience & persistence. Make sure the pictures you add to your portfolio are high-quality images - preferably taken by a professional photographer.

The best way to start is by volunteering your makeup services to local wedding photographers, friends & family. Let them know you're willing to do a free trial/consultation and makeup on the actual day. In return for your free services ask for some wedding pictures for your portfolio. Keep volunteering until you feel your portfolio has enough images that showcase your range of skills.

Where you can find local wedding photographers

Local wedding photographers are commonly found on wedding planning and directory guides websites like:

- Mywedding.com
- Projectwedding.com
- Theknot.com
- Thumbtack.com
- Weddingwire.com
- Yelp.com

Other places:

- Yellow Pages
- Google search (type wedding photographers + your city/town)

Portfolio Alternative

If you have trouble finding a photographer or none of your friends/family are getting married at the moment, you can create a simple "before & after" portfolio. This portfolio should have before and after shots of 5-10 women. Ask your family/friends if they can volunteer.

When taking any "before" shots, make sure the women look really plain (hair undone, wearing a T-shirt, etc). When taking any "after" shots, make sure their hair is styled nicely to suit the makeup. Also consider what they are wearing – perhaps they can bring a nice dress to wear (if they have a wedding dress even better). Focus on taking pictures from the shoulder up rather than full body shots. Be sure that you get close-ups of the face too. Look at other bridal portfolios for posing ideas.

Avoid taking pictures in direct sunlight. The light is too strong and will wash out your subject. Always try to take pictures by a window where sunlight is being filtered through a sheer white curtain. The light will be soft and flattering and your pictures will look more professional. If you need more help please do an online search for: how to take good pictures or diy professional photos. We also encourage you to use editing software to brighten or crop your photos as needed. Great and free editing software can be found at Picasa.com and Picmonkey.com

Helpful Tips

- When you are applying makeup to a real bride, make sure to write down the products & colors you applied at the trial/consultation. Paper or digital makeup charts are useful to keep track of this information. You can also take a picture of the bride so you can refer back to the exact makeup application.

- Encourage the bride to bring photo of what she likes. This will help you get an idea of how soft or strong her makeup should be.

- Heavily touched-up pictures can look fake and be misleading. Avoid adding any to your portfolio.

- Keep your portfolio fresh and up to date by replacing old photos with newer ones.

- Maintain professionalism at all times even while you are not getting paid.

- Do not Tweet or post pictures on Facebook while you're working. Posting images or tagging without people's permission can tarnish your reputation!

- Always ask the owner of the photos for permission to use the photos.

- Keep track of the names of the photographers you work with. You never know when you may need a letter of recommendation or reference.

25 Jumpstarting Your Career

Jumpstarting a career in the personal beauty service industry begins with self-promotion. Self-promotion is about getting the word out about your services *to the right people*. Being able to promote yourself is honestly just as important as knowing how to apply makeup. The key to successful self-promotion begins with the right tools. To get started, you will need the following:

- Business cards
- Brochures
- Portfolio

Business cards

You want your business cards to be eye-catching and unique. Zazzle.com is an excellent source for customizable cards with designs geared towards makeup artists (enter makeup artist in the search bar on zazzle.com). Moo.com is a great source for full size cards or mini-cards that you can customize with images from your portfolio.

Brochures

Brochures are great for showcasing images from your portfolio. Be sure to include your rate/pricing, a menu of the services you offer, whether you travel to customers or not, web address & your contact information. Websites that offer customizable brochures templates & printing services include: Uprinting.com, Vistaprint.com, 123print.com and Print.staples.com.

Flyers & post cards are great alternatives to brochures. You'll find most of these sites also offer customizable flyers & post card templates.

Portfolio

In the personal beauty service industry a hard copy portfolio is equally important as a digital one. Sometimes, when meeting in person with potential customers or clients, its a lot easier to show your hard copy "book" than it is get online to show your digital one. However, when you are just starting, a digital portfolio will be the most useful in terms of self-promotion. You can have a digital portfolio up & running in minutes with a website builder or through a social website like modelmayhem.com, makeupart.net or bloom.com.

Most website builders and social websites offer "free" or "subscription" based options. Although free may sound like a great bargain, be aware that there is a downside. Basically with a free website, you do not own your own web address (URL). The website builder will choose a URL for you and usually it'll be one that's long & hard to remember.

You want to be able to use your web address on other marketing materials so it needs to be as memorable as possible. Generally a "subscription" based option will allow you to choose your own web address for a monthly fee.

In addition to displaying images, a digital portfolio should also be used to share important information about your business & yourself. Whenever possible, fill out or create the following sections:

About

Use this section to "brag" about yourself. Be honest about your strengths/skills, why you're passionate about doing makeup & why you're the perfect person for the job. You should also include a professional looking picture of yourself.

Services

The services section should include menu of the services you offer. You should also list your pricing/rates & whether you travel to clients or not.

Contact

Let you prospective clients know how to reach you. Make sure your contact information stays up to date. Use Gmail, Yahoo or another email provider to create a free email specifically for your makeup business. You can also use this email address on your business and comp-card.

In addition to having your own site, you can also place your portfolio on wedding planning sites & local guides like weddingwire.com, mywedding.com, theknot.com, weddingvibe.com, yelp.com and thumbtack.com (sign up as a "vendor"). These sites expose your work to brides & other wedding related professionals searching for makeup services.

How to Start Promoting Yourself

The quickest way to reach your potential clients is through wedding planning & local guide websites. These sites provide a great opportunity for you to expose your digital portfolio to people searching for makeup services. It's free to sign up and your portfolio will be online within a matter of hours. (Make sure you sign up as a "vendor" or "service provider).

Popular wedding planning and local guide sites are:

- Mywedding.com
- Theknot.com
- Thumbtack.com
- Weddingvibe.com
- Weddingwire.com
- Yelp.com

SCAM ALERT!!!

Online makeup artist communities have reported scams that target makeup artists. They warn of people who contact you by email and want to book you for services. This "client" says they want to pay you "up front". They ask for your mailing address to send you check. Once you receive their fake check "worth" thousands of dollars, the scammers then tell you they over paid you by "accident". They then ask you to deposit the check into your bank account and wire the money back right away (without waiting for the check to clear).Those who fall for this scam actually wire thousands of dollars of their own money and then come to find out the check was fake or bounced. Don't be another victim! Beware of emails that talk about paying you up front and that come from someone who doesn't want to talk to you on the phone/person.

Network with others that service the bride

Building solid relationships with others that service the bride can also help you reach potential clients. Other service providers include:

- Bridal Shops/Boutiques
- Salons/Hair Stylists
- Wedding Photographers
- Wedding Planners

You easily find these service providers through the same wedding planning & local guide sites mentioned above. A local online search will provide you more names. Make initial contact through a friendly email (leave a link to your portfolio-website). Whenever possible go to a service provider's office or place of business to introduce yourself in person. Another great place meet others is at bridal fairs and shows. Be sure you leave your business card and/or some brochures card with everyone you meet. Remember to always start and end a conversation on an upbeat note.

Let word of mouth work for you

You'd surprised how quickly your business can grow from people spreading the word about you. Start by letting all your friends and family know you're doing makeup. Offer free makeup trails so they get a chance to see your skills and expertise. Give everyone a few cards/brochures that they can hand out to others in need of your services.

Give back to your community

Offer women in your community free makeup demonstrations/makeovers. This will give you a chance to connect to people outside of your friends/family. It also helps you earn the trust and respect of others when they see you giving back to the community. All you basically need to start is a small foldable table (to place business cards, brochures & your hard copy portfolio), a makeup/directors chair and your makeup kit. Make sure you speak to the manager to ask for permission & make arrangements. Good places to try are:

- Women's gyms
- Nursing homes
- Shelters for abused women
- Bridal Boutiques

Build Referral Clientele

Make conversation with others when you're out shopping or running errands. Give each new contact 2 business cards. Ask them to keep a card for themselves and share the other card with someone they know who could use your services.

Self-Promotion Tip

Utilize social networks like to connect, interact and maintain communication with people you meet. These social platforms are great for sharing images from your portfolio and linking to your website. Popular sites include:

- Facebook.com
- Pinterest.com
- Foursquare.com
- Google+.com
- Myspace.com
- Tumblr.com
- Twitter.com

Conclusion

Self-promotion is all about getting the word out that you exist & that you have something to offer. In order for it to be effective you must connect with people *who need your services*. Don't forget makeup artistry is a PEOPLE BUSINESS. A positive and humble attitude can open many doors of opportunities for you!

Chapter 7
Getting Started In Media Production

In This Chapter:

- How Productions Work
- The Role of an Agency
- What is a Union Production?
- Building Essential Skills
- Building a Portfolio
- Jumpstarting Your Career

26 How Productions Work

Productions run on budgets and schedules. The budget determines how much money is allotted for costs including makeup services. A production schedule is broken down into 3 phases:

Phase 1: Pre-production

- Planning, development & preparation stage. Cast and crew are hired.

Phase 2: Production

- Actual shooting/filming/performance takes place. The makeup artist will prepare touch up and remove makeup from talent as required throughout this time.

Phase 3: Post-production

- Editing takes place. Final release and distribution occurs after this process. Usually the lengthiest part of the production process.

Budgets and the length of time of a production schedule vary per project. Also the daily work schedule can vary. Typically, photo and video shoots run a few days while movies, TV and theater tend to take the most time to produce- extending weeks, months or even years in some cases.

27 The Role of an Agency

Many media makeup artists turn to agencies for representation, management and career guidance/support. In addition to presenting your work to potential clients, agencies take care of other duties on your behalf such as:

- Negotiate pay rates & work terms
- Bills/invoices the production co.
- Handles money coming in
- Marketing and promotions

In exchange for their services, agencies charge their makeup artists a percentage of their earnings. Generally it's around 10-20%.

There are a few key elements to get signed with an agency. First and foremost, your portfolio must reflect quality work. Remember quality over quantity. Usually 10 strong images are enough to show an agency your range of talent and skills. Is very important that your portfolio is something the agency will want to show their clients. Look at the portfolios of the makeup artists they currently represent, this will give you a good idea of what they are looking for. The second crucial element is your personality. Agencies want to make sure your easy to work with, have a positive attitude and will make a good impression on their clients.

Many makeup artists have found representation by assisting a makeup artist who is signed with agency. Although you may work for free at first, building a professional relationship with another makeup artist is priceless. Knowing they can count on you can lead to future recommendations to their agency and their clients.

It's important to note that there are unethical agencies that exist. If an agency ever asks for money up front from you, it's probably a scam. Legitimate agencies work on commission. If you ever feel unsure about an agency, check with the Better Business Bureau (bbb.org) or RipoffReport.com.

ADDITIONAL RESOURCES

To learn more about preparing yourself for an agency we recommend:

Crystal Wright is the owner of Crystal Agency and represents many celebrity makeup artists. She is also an educator who has published:

- Crystal Wright's 1-Day Portfolio Building Workshop 4-DVDs
- Crystal Wrights Hair Makeup & Fashion Styling Career Guide

Available on amazon.com or thestore.crystalwrightlive.com

28   What Is A Union Production?

A union is an organization that represents workers to ensure they receive fair treatment in the work force. They negotiate wages/rates, working conditions, health benefits and pensions. It also serves as a source for industry news, trade events and continuing education.

The International Alliance of Theatrical Stage Employees (IATSE) is a union or guild that was formed by freelancing artisans and technicians working in motion picture and stage. The most well known division of IATSE is Local 706 — which represents makeup artists as well as hair stylists in Hollywood, California. The IATSE has expanded to represent makeup artists working in:

- live theater
- motion picture
- television productions
- trade shows and exhibitions,
- concerts
- video/digital media

The IASTE can be found throughout the US and Canada. While the IASTE is the most recognized union that exists, there are others in the US and internationally. Each local office determines the requirements on how to become a member. Generally those requirements include proof of experience in production and a registration fee (which can range from hundreds to thousands of dollars). Once accepted as a member, a makeup artist is responsible for attending meetings & paying dues – including a percentage of their wages to the IASTE.

Productions that are considered "union" are under contract with a union. Generally union production co. only hire from a roster of union workers/members. However, if there is a shortage of union workers or if a director/talent specifically requests a non-union makeup artist, a production co. has been known to hire non-union workers. In these cases, the production co. is required by law to provide the same benefits to a non-union worker that a union worker would receive. Often because of this, the non-union artist is required to pay a percentage of their wages to the union for "reaping" the benefits of a union job.

At times, union members may find work on a production that is non-union. In "Right to Work" states the makeup artist should have option to take a job with no restrictions. While in "Union" states the worker may face a penalty accepting the job. Understanding the rules of the union will ultimately determine if there would be a repercussion.

Research reveals unconfirmed reports of non-union makeup artists pressured to join unions or face blacklisting from future productions. While there are many who value and appreciate the efforts unions to keep jobs in the hands of their members, others strongly disagree with any tactics to intimidate non-members or disrupt productions that choose to work with non-union makeup artists.

These pressing issues and controversy have contributed to "runaway productions". These fleeing productions relocate in order to reduce production costs & separate themselves from the bureaucracy of unions and big studio systems. Another big factor for relocating has been due to tax breaks and incentives offered by other states and even other countries. One of the world's leading entertainment capitals, Los Angeles California, has been the most impacted by this change.

29   Building Essential Skills

If you decide you'd like to pursue a career in media production, it's crucial to gain the right skills. There are several options when it comes to training. You might decide to attend a makeup school or consider alterative learning tools/training resources. Which ever training option you decide to go with, it's important to understand which skills you need to build.

One of the best training sources for building essential skills is to assist a professional makeup artist. While you may not get apply makeup right away, you can learn a lot by watching and listening to someone with experience. Start by contacting an artist directly. Let them know you're interested in learning and would like to offer your assistance free of charge. Excellent sources to find pro artist in your area are:

- Hmartistsnetwork.com
- Makeup talent agencies
- Modelmayhem.com
- yelp.com

In addition to assisting an artist, you can also hire a makeup artist to be your personal mentor/coach. Excellent sources to find makeup artists who want to mentor beginners:

- Makeuplessons.com
- Makeupmentors.com
- Hmartistsnetwork.com/one-on-one-apprenticing

List of Essential Skills

Essential media production skills fall into 6 categories:

- Safe Beauty
- History of Beauty

- Beauty Makeup
- Beyond Beauty Makeup*
- Technical Media
- Business

Safe Beauty Skills

The first skills you must acquire are disease control and prevention aka safe beauty skills. As we previously discussed, it may be required by law for you to obtain a cosmetology license. Please refer back to *Chapter 4 - Makeup Artist Licensing-* for more information and instructions.

History of Beauty

It's important to be able to create realistic historical looks if a production calls for it, so a media makeup artist must have an accurate sense of how people appeared throughout ancient and contemporary history. Here are a few books that can help you gain knowledge on this subject.

- Fashions in Makeup: From Ancient to Modern Times by Richard Corson

- The Artifice of Beauty: A History and Practical Guide to Perfume and Cosmetics by Sally Pointer

- History of Compacts and Cosmetics: From Victorian Times to the Present Day by Madeleine Marsh, amazon.com

All available on amazon.com

Beauty Makeup Skills

Beauty makeup skills are the most essential and common skills used by makeup artists in media production. Focus on learning the following types of Beauty styles:

- Clean beauty
- Basic beauty
- Fashion
- Glamour
- High Fashion

Beyond Beauty Skills

If you're interested in theater, television and/or movies you'll also need to learn character/special effects makeup in addition to beauty makeup.

Technical Media Skills

Technical Media skills are necessary to be able to apply makeup for cameras and a variety of lighting conditions. Here are a few learning tools that can help you gain knowledge on this subject.

- The Makeup Artist Handbook: Techniques for Film, Television, Photography and Theatre by Gretchen Davis and Mindy Hall

- Graftobian HD Makeup 101 - Achieving Perfection with Simplicity DVD

- Airbrush Makeup 101 DVD by Temptu

Business Skills

Business skills are essential to for managing and growing your business. Most importantly, they will prepare you for providing quality professional service to your clients. Business skills for media production involve the following:

- Self- Employed/Freelancer
- Sales & Customer Service

Self- Employed/Freelancer skills allow you run a business whether you decide to work in a salon/spa based or as a mobile makeup artist. These skills include setting up a business, how to negotiate your rates, creating contracts and invoices, managing your finances, filing your taxes, obtaining personal/liability insurance & finding work through marketing and self-promotion.

Customer Service & Sales skills are essential in dealing with people and conveying the right message about your services. When applied correctly, these skills will earn you loyal lifetime clients and a strong referral base.

To help you get started building business skills for the media production industry, we recommend:

- The Hair Makeup & Fashion Styling Career Guide, 5th Edition by Crystal Wright

- Visit HMArtistsnetwork.com for their planning guide

30   Building a Portfolio

Once you've had time to develop your skills to work in media production, you can start building a portfolio. A portfolio is the most important promotional tool for a media makeup artist. If you choose to acquire training through a makeup school, you'll want to find out if the school will assist you in building one. If they do not or if you choose not attend a school this section will get you started.

In the media industry it's common to find photographers and other creative professionals "testing" to build their portfolios. A "test" is essentially a photo shoot where everyone involves donates their time and talent in exchange for photos. Another term for testing is TFP which means "test for print" or "trade for print".

During a test or TFP you can find photographers, models, hairstylists, wardrobe stylists & makeup artists volunteer their time and services. They all come together to collaborate for the purpose of capturing a portfolio-worthy image.

How to Start Testing

Before you can begin its important to understand that some photographers may want to see some of your work before they consider testing with you. Since the whole point of testing is to get some images what can you do?

You'll need to find a professional photographer who is willing to give you a chance. Let the photographer know you're just getting started and would like an opportunity to start building your portfolio. When looking for photographers to test with, it's always best to check out their portfolio first. Make sure their style of photography is what you would like to see in your portfolio.

Where to find photographers:

- Modelmayhem.com
- Photography/Art School with photography programs
- Modeling agencies - photographers are always testing with new models.
- Hair and Makeup Agencies - agencies usually have a test list that they send out when photographers need to test.
- Find names of photographers in the credits of local magazines.
- Google search
- Yellow Pages

Of all the resources just mentioned, we highly advise you to consider using modelmayhem.com. On modelmayhem.com you'll find established photographers with connections to models as well as stylist who may also want to test.

 When you find a photographer to test with you awesome! Next, find out when they will be ready to shoot and make sure it fits in your schedule. You'll also need to discuss:

- Time & Location
- Who will be the model
- Hairstylist
- Wardrobe stylist
- Ideas about the theme (colors, makeup style, hair style, clothes, etc…)*
- How long does post-editing take?(Photoshop touchups, cropping the photos, etc)
- Where and how photos will be delivered (usually sent by email)

* Creating a theme for test shoot is a team effort. If you have great ideas or a concept in mind, speak up. And don't forget to listen to the concepts/ideas of others involved too.

To get the most of out of a test, be sure to ask the photographer for:

- As many close up shots of the makeup as possible
- Photos that aren't heavily touched up. This can look fake & misleading.
- 2 – 3 makeup changes if time permits-build your portfolio quicker!

After you receive the photos from the shoot, add them to your portfolio. Keep on building your portfolio by testing with better and better photographers. Use every test shoot as an opportunity to add another image that will show your range of makeup skills.

Tips for Testing

- When you're at a photo shoot, be mindful of photography equipment - it is very expensive! Don't have food and drinks or things than can potentially ruin the equipment. Also watch your step.

- Be mindful of stepping in front of the camera for a touch up. Let the photographer know you are doing so.

- See how the makeup you applied is reading on camera by doing a "camera test". After seeing how the makeup looks you can make any necessary adjustments.

- Stay for the entire shoot. A photographer appreciates and sees that you care. You want to be sure you're present so you can make corrections and/or changes as needed.

- Keep gum or mints with you to keep your breath fresh. Also take a healthy snack and drink if the test is going to last several hours.

- Do not Tweet or post pictures on Facebook while you're working. Posting images or tagging without people's permission can tarnish your reputation! This applies for tests and actual paying jobs!!

- Be prepared to travel. Sometimes a photographer may want to take some pictures at different locations. Have a set bag ready to go with makeup you will need.

- Help the photographer. He/she may need help with light reflectors and/or other equipment. The more help you can be the better the picture you will get for your portfolio. It also helps build a sense of teamwork.

- Maintain professionalism at all times even while you are not getting paid. The impression you leave the model or photographer may lead to paying jobs in the future if they remember you as reliable, a great attitude, easy to work with and lots of talent.

- Keep track of the names of the photographers you test with. You can start to build your resume with those names of. You also never know when you may need a letter of recommendation or reference.

- Keep track of all your test shoots photos. Photographers can be very busy and forget to send them to you. A friendly email is a nice way to remind them.

- Makeup sure you have the owner of the pictures permission to use the images (usually the photographer is the owner).

ADDITIONAL RESOURCES

To learn more about building a professional portfolio for the media production industry we've gathered the following resources to help you.

- Packaging Your Portfolio & Marketing Live Workshop
- 1-Day Portfolio Building Workshop 4-DVDs
- The Hair, Makeup & Styling Career Guide, 5th Edition

Available at thestore.crystalwrightlive.com & amazon.com.

Model Mayhem Forum

Learn from and join the conversation with other pro makeup artists & industry professionals. There's a wealth of information you can find about portfolios, testing, photo shoots & more. Visit modelmayhem.com

31 Jumpstarting Your Career

Jumpstarting a career in the media production industry begins with self-promotion. Self-promotion is about getting the word out about your services *to the right people*. Being able to promote yourself is honestly just as important as knowing how to apply makeup. The key to successful self-promotion begins with the right tools. To get started you will need the following:

- Business cards
- Comp cards
- Portfolio

Business cards

You want your business cards to be eye-catching and unique. Zazzle.com is an excellent source for customizable cards with designs geared towards makeup artists (enter makeup artist in the search bar on zazzle.com). Moo.com is a great source for full size cards or mini-cards that you can customize with images from your portfolio.

Comp cards

A comp card or zed card is essentially a fancy flyer you can handout. It's used to showcase images from your portfolio & provide your contact information. Websites such as Compcardprinter.com, Theprintcollective.com, Compcardexpress.com & Printing4today.com offer comp card printing services.

Please note: most comp cards templates are designed for actors and models but can be customized to suit a makeup artist.

Portfolio

In media production a hard copy portfolio is equally important as a digital one. When meeting with production companies or agencies, they may ask to see your "book". However, when you are just starting, a digital portfolio will be the most useful. You can have a digital portfolio up & running in minutes with a website builder or through a social website like modelmayhem.com, makeupart.net or bloom.com.

Most website builders and social websites offer "free" or "subscription" based options. Although free may sound like a great bargain, be aware that there is a downside. Basically with a free website, you do not own your own web address (URL). The website builder will choose a URL for you and usually it'll be one that's long & hard to remember.

You want to be able to use your web address on other your other promotion/marketing material, so it needs to be easy to remember. Generally a "subscription" based option will allow you to choose your own web address for a monthly fee.

In addition to displaying your photos, a digital portfolio can also be used to share important information about yourself. Whenever possible fill out or create a section for the following:

About

Use this section to "brag" about yourself. Be honest about your strengths/skills, why you're passionate about doing makeup & why you're the perfect person for the job. You should also include a professional looking picture of yourself.

Credits

The "credits" section gives people visiting your website a quick look at your professional experience. You'll want to list all the professional photographers you've tested/worked with. Update it every so often to add any new ones to the list. Also, list names of production companies once you start working.

Contact

Let prospective clients know how to reach you. Make sure your contact information stays up to date. Use Gmail, Yahoo or another email provider to create a free email specifically for your makeup business. You can also use this email address on your business and comp-card.

How to Start Promoting Yourself

Once your portfolio-website is ready to go, you can start targeting the type of production(s) you're interested in. You can find local production co. in your area by doing an online search. Call or send them an email to find out about future projects and who's in charge of hiring. Send them a link to your website-portfolio.

Help your clients find you

Another important element of self-promotion is making it easy for people to find you. Productions often turn to network/directory/talent listing sites in search of makeup artists. Many of these sites allow you to search through casting calls and job openings posted by production companies. Utilize sites like:

- Modelhayem.com
- Makeupart.net
- HMArtistsnetwork.com
- Makeupartistjobs.com
- Thepowdergroup.com
- Models.com
- Onemodelplace.com
- Productionhub.com
- Variety411.com

If you are not able to add images from your portfolio to these directory sites, be sure link to your website-portfolio so people can still see your work.

SCAM ALERT!!!

Online makeup artist communities have reported scams that target makeup artists. They warn of people who contact you by email and want to book you for services. This "client" says they want to pay you "up front". They ask for your mailing address to send you check. Once you receive their fake check "worth" thousands of dollars, the scammers then tell you they over paid you by "accident". They then ask you to deposit the check into your bank account and wire the money back right away (without waiting for the check to clear).Those who fall for this scam actually wire thousands of dollars of their own money and then come to find out the check was fake or bounced. Don't be another victim! Beware of emails that talk about paying you up front and that come from someone who doesn't want to talk to you on the phone/person.

Face to Face Connections

Attend industry events related to the production(s) you're interested in. Leave your business card or comp card with people you make contact with. Remember to always start and end a conversation on an upbeat note.

Assist a Makeup Artist

Another great way to get your foot in the door is by assisting a key makeup artist. Assisting allows you gain experience, build professional relationships and make new connections. You never know who you'll meet on a production that may need a makeup artist for a future project. Start by contacting a working professional makeup artist. Let them know you're interested in learning and would like to offer your assistance free of charge. Send them a link to your website so they know you're serious. Excellent sources to find pro artist in your area are:

- Modelmayhem.com
- Hmartistsnetwork.com
- Yelp.com
- Makeup talent agencies

Self-Promotion Tip

Utilize social networks like to connect, interact and maintain communication with people you meet. These social platforms are great for sharing images from your portfolio and linking to your website. Popular sites include:

- Facebook.com
- Pinterest.com
- Foursquare.com
- Google+.com
- Modelmayhem.com
- Myspace.com
- Tumblr.com
- Twitter.com

Conclusion

Self-promotion is all about getting the word out that you exist & that you have something to offer. In order for it to be effective, you must connect with people *who need your services*. Don't forget makeup artistry is a PEOPLE BUSINESS. A positive and humble attitude can open many doors of opportunities for you!

ADDITIONAL RESOURCES

To learn more about self-promotion in the media industry we recommend you read:

- Crystal Wrights Hair Makeup & Fashion Styling Career Guide

Available on amazon.com & thestore.crystalwrightlive.com

Visit out online directory guide at www.careersinmakeup.com
for links to resources mentioned in this book.

5677672R00079

Made in the USA
San Bernardino, CA
16 November 2013